I'm Still Sexy
So What's Up with Him?

I'm Still Sexy
So What's Up
with Him?

Learn How Testosterone
Can Change Your Relationship

Sloan Teeple M.D. *&* Susan Teeple

NEW YORK

I'm Still Sexy So What's Up with Him?
Learn How Testosterone Can Change Your Relationship

ISBN 978-1-61448-219-2 paperback
ISBN 978-1-61448-220-8 eBook
Library of Congress Control Number: 2012932320

Morgan James Publishing
The Entrepreneurial Publisher
5 Penn Plaza, 23rd Floor,
New York City, New York 10001
(212) 655-5470 office • (516) 908-4496 fax
www.MorganJamesPublishing.com

Cover Design by:
Rachel Lopez
www.r2cdesign.com

Interior Design by:
Bonnie Bushman
bonnie@caboodlegraphics.com

In an effort to support local communities, raise awareness and funds, Morgan James Publishing donates a percentage of all book sales for the life of each book to Habitat for Humanity Peninsula and Greater Williamsburg.

Get involved today, visit
www.MorganJamesBuilds.com.

To our precious children,
Chase, Hudson and Evelyn Teeple

Table of Contents

CHAPTER ONE   I'm still sexy, so what's wrong with him?   1

CHAPTER TWO   It's OK to Laugh   9

CHAPTER THREE   The Signs and Symptoms of Low T   19

CHAPTER FOUR   Broaching the Subject   33

CHAPTER FIVE   What Can We Do?   47

CHAPTER SIX   How Can We Find a Doctor?   59

CHAPTER SEVEN   What Should We Expect?   65

CHAPTER EIGHT   Who's At Risk?   73

CHAPTER NINE   A Wonder Drug …
or Just Good Medicine?   91

CHAPTER TEN   What about Prostate Cancer?   107

CHAPTER ELEVEN   What About Getting Older?   119

CHAPTER TWELVE   What If We Don't Get Treatment?   129

CHAPTER THIRTEEN Your Role, Ladies   139

CHAPTER FOURTEEN Q & A   151

Conclusion   155

Author Biography   157

Acknowledgements

I'm Still Sexy So What's Up With Him has been a culmination of years of medical training, practice, personal struggle and triumph, and life-expieriences. You would not be seeing these words in print if it was not for our friend and consultant: Dr. Scott Sticksel. Thanks to his encouragement and connections we have given birth to this book. He protected, guided, and inspired us every step of the way. Scott introduced us to the gifted writer Steve Halliday, who helped us put our life experience onto paper. We will be forever grateful to Scott and Steve's commitment to seeing this project to completion.

We owe a special thanks to the extraordinary Rick Schirmer, of DBA Worldwide, who has taken us under his wing and inspired us with his energy, imagination and creativity. Brandon Piety, Christine Saleh, and Dillon Wilson, who has graciously worked on this project, thank you for your enthusiasm. It was a joy to work with Cameron Cone, and his wife Jacquelyn, to capture the images for this book. You are a truly talented "ninja" of the photography world. To David Hancock, Margo Toulouse and Bethany Marshall and all our friends at Morgan James Publishing: thank you for your professionalism and trust in us and this book.

In the academic arena, there are no greater champions for testosterone deficiency awareness and treatment than Dr. Larry Lipshultz, Dr. Abraham Morgentaler and Dr. Irwin Goldstein. What we know about testosterone is in large part due to their research and dedication to this field. I am grateful to them for sharing their knoweledge and expierence with me, as well as the generous gift of their time. To my seven medical partners at Amarillo Urology Associates, thank you all for your encouragement and patience during this project. It is a joy to practice medicine with you all. My office staff is an extraordinary group of individuals, and I could not have done this book without them. Chris, Arthur, Rudy, and Laura work with me day in and day out, and help me provide the best care possible to my patients. Thanks for your hard work and for keeping me smiling and on track. Finally, thank you to my patients, especially the ones who generously shared their personal stories for this book – I am in your debt. You have done a great service to men and women by allowing me to share your story in this book.

Our friends and family, to whom we owe more than we can possibly say, we could not have gotten to this point if it were not for your love and encouragement. Especially Spencer and Aaron for their wise counsel and sharing of their thoughts throughout this process. Many thanks to Jo Sevier who holds down the fort and keeps us smiling. To our grandmother Ibby Hardie, who is always sending us articles and newsclippings and is the hippest 90 year old we know: we love you. Our parents have always believed in us and have given us the confidence to share the good, bad and our true life story. We hope we have made you proud.

Last but certainly not least, to the three loves of our life: our children Chase, Hudson and Evie. You have our deepest gratitude, love and respect.

I'm Still Sexy, So What's Wrong with Him?

For the longest time, Susan couldn't figure out what was wrong. She figured the problem somehow had to be her fault. Why didn't I seem interested in her physically? Why had sex fallen so far down on my list of things to do?

We'd been married about a dozen years, had two young sons, and led a stressful life navigating a medical residency. But while Susan could handle my jam-packed schedule, she anguished over my lack of desire for intimacy—especially after I showed zero interest when she expressed a strong desire to try for a daughter.

That devastated her.

Until that point, she had noted my increasingly somber moods, my preference to be alone, and my general lack of energy, but had attributed it all to the rigors of becoming a physician. She thought the long hours and frequent exhaustion simply had to be accepted as the steep price for admission to the medical community. And while it bothered her that I seemed to lack interest in sex, she thought, *Well, I already have a four-year-old and a two-year-old. I'm not that* interested in sex, either. It's not like I'm walking around in lingerie all the time.*

My utterly indifferent response to her clearly expressed desire to have another child, however—well, that bothered her. A lot.

Like many women, Susan immediately blamed herself. She took herself through a long and deeply self-incriminating list of possible reasons for our predicament. *OK, she thought. I've lost all my baby weight. I work out all the time. My hair looks really pretty. So what's wrong with me?* She assumed that our problem had to be her problem, and so for a long time she looked for an answer within herself. She mentally played out all the possible scenarios to explain her part in turning me off sexually. Her weight? No. Her appearance? No. Her hygiene? No. Her education? No. Could I be having an affair? She knew me better than that. The questions kept coming, but so did the negative responses.

Over time she began wondering if any of these "explanations" held water. After another extended period of painful self-grilling, she concluded, quite rightly, *"There's nothing wrong with me. The problem has got to be with **him**."*

Eventually the day came when she felt she had to talk it out with me. She approached me, pointed to her shapely body, and said, *"Sloan, look at me. I've been working so hard. This is as good as it gets. If you're not attracted to this, then you need to know it's only going to go downhill from here."*

Her words startled me, but I replied deliberately and with a slow shake of my head. "Susan," I declared, "it's not you"—but of course, she already knew that. I had hoped my humble response would end the discussion, but thankfully, it didn't. Susan looked me square in the eyes and then hit me with another query, in fact, The Question. Maybe if I had prepared for it, I could have fended it off. But she caught me unprepared, and so it took me completely by surprise.

"Are you gay?"

My jaw dropped even as my head spun around. What did she just ask? I'm not gay, of course, but that's the last question I ever expected to hear from my dear wife. Had things deteriorated so much in our lives together that she had begun to seriously question my sexuality?

I'm grateful that Susan is no wallflower. God used her shocking question to move me out of my rut and get me started on the road toward health and wholeness.

Immediately I scheduled myself for a complete physical checkup. I don't recall exactly what I expected to find, but the results gave me another shock. After the tests came back, the doctor pronounced me in excellent health—except for one thing.

"You have the testosterone level of an eighty-year-old man," he said. And I had not yet celebrated my thirty-third birthday!

I learned on that unforgettable day that I had a testosterone level of under 200, a figure so low that doctors expected to see it only in seniors half a century my elders (since then, medical science has shifted its opinion; today, doctors believe a healthy eighty-year-old man should have a testosterone level of about 300, or more than a hundred points higher than mine when I first got tested!).

Most surprising of all, perhaps, I had no clue about any of this— and if anyone should have had a clue, it was me. After all, I had studied hard for many long years to become a urologist, a glorified plumber. If any medical doctor should know about testosterone problems, it's a urology resident. But like nearly all of my colleagues, I had received almost no training in diagnosing or treating low testosterone and the life-altering problems that such a condition can provoke. I simply didn't know that my sex drive wasn't where it was supposed to be. The loss of libido had come gradually and both Susan and I had attributed it to the stressors of a high-pressure medical residency.

We were wrong.

Sometime later I learned that Susan had noticed a number of disquieting changes in me that had taken place over a period of many months. She recognized something had gone wrong, but couldn't quite put her finger on it. Yet while she noted the changes, none of them really alarmed her . . . until they began destroying our sex lives. I had become more isolated, less outgoing, more tired, less engaged with our boys. I almost never laughed. I lacked almost all drive and motivation and had grown disinterested in outside activities that I once found enjoyable. The serious side of me had taken over and produced a world-class Stoic. In a word, Susan told me, "Sloan, you lost your mojo." I had become a different person from the man she had married, and she wanted the old Sloan back.

Susan and I still laugh about the time, before my diagnosis, that two good friends threw a dinner party for my birthday. After our meal and during the dessert, I fell fast asleep . . . right at the dinner table. I nodded off, leaving three puzzled and wide-awake adults wondering what had happened. And understand this incident took place after I had become a senior resident, which meant I was getting more sleep than I had enjoyed for many months before.

So with diagnosis in hand, about five years ago I began testosterone replacement therapy. I started out with injections, then moved to a gel (we'll talk about these options later). I saw almost immediate results. Within two or three days, my libido kicked in. I started looking forward to playing with my kids. Physical exercise began producing marked results in my body, unlike before. I gained fresh focus and found renewed energy. I had grown so used to feeling tired that I had almost forgotten the feeling of being so alive!

Susan began recognizing the benefits of my treatment within a few months. She said the core things that make me "me" came back again. I became more vital, more alive. I grew more spontaneous, more daring. And our love life reawakened from the dead.

Evie, our daughter, is now six years old.

Today, I'm enjoying life like never before. That doesn't mean, of course, that testosterone therapy is a magical cure; it's not. Nor is it a fountain of youth. But for a huge number of guys (and the women who love them), restoring a healthy testosterone level can be the secret to renewed mental, physical, and sexual well-being. The Federal Drug Administration estimated about five years ago that 15 million men in America had low testosterone. While I think that number is significantly low, consider that only five percent of those 15 million men are ever diagnosed. That means that at least 14.25 million American men—and probably many millions more—suffer from low testosterone and its life-hampering consequences without even knowing it.

That's why I decided to write this book.

And that's why we've written it.

The Crucial Role of Women

Hardly a week goes by in my urology practice that I don't get introduced to a man who suffers from medically low levels of testosterone. But almost never does he walk into my office of his own accord. Nearly always a wife or fiancee or girlfriend or other significant woman in his life has urged him to get tested for "something." Like my wife, these women can't quite put their finger on the problem; but the changes they've seen overtake their men worry them and prompt them to urge their loved ones to "go see the doctor."

Thank God for such women! They often observe and note with concern what completely escapes us as men. Without their proactive intervention—something that many oblivious males don't always appreciate—we'd continue to descend further and further into isolation, exhaustion, general apathy and an increasing lack of joy. We certainly would miss out on becoming all we can be, which I think ought to be a top goal for all of us. I like what Susan (my "not a wallflower" partner) says:

I don't think it's OK to accept mediocrity. Life has its peaks and valleys, of course, but I dislike it when I hear people our age complain about various physical problems and chalk it up to "aging." Maybe it is, and maybe it isn't. I think people need to live life to the fullest, to find God's plan for them and then fulfill it. And you're not going to do that in front of the TV, depressed and sad. You're going to do it by getting out in the world.

Sloan's not particularly thrilled to let people know that he had erection problems when he was thirty-two years old, or that he had the testosterone of an eighty-year-old. But we believe that by telling our story, more people can learn how to thrive. Like everyone else, we have to go out of our comfort zone to live the life God has for us. People have a hard time keeping up with Sloan now, because he's full of energy. Sometimes he looks so focused and energetic that he makes the rest of the world look like it's moving v-e-r-y s-l-o-w-l-y.

While I can't vouch for all of Susan's observations, she believes, as I do, that we are stewards of each other's health. We're in this battle together. Sometimes I put calcium tablets on the table for her to take, and sometimes she notices a change in me that warrants a checkup.

So with this crucial dynamic in mind, we decided to write this book together. While I'll be writing from a medical perspective, Susan will be writing from a steward's perspective—as a partner and member of Team Teeple. When we write as a unit or I write from my own perspective, the text will appear as it does now.

And when Susan writes from her unique perspective, the type font will change to reflect her style.

We hope in this way to bring you a balanced, multi-perspective, team-oriented approach to dealing with the problems of low testosterone. Throughout this book, we hope to give you the best, most up-to-date information available on the medical aspects of the issue, as well as provide you with helpful, real-world counsel on what to expect, how to proceed, and pitfalls to avoid.

In order to make this work as useful to you as possible, we've also solicited the help of a number of other couples who are on this same journey. We've interviewed men and women about their own experience with low testosterone and asked them to share ideas, practices, and insights that they have found beneficial—as well as approaches that haven't worked quite so well. We've tried, in other words, to combine the best and most current medical thinking on this challenge with the wisdom of real men and women who deal with it every day. As much as possible, we want to bring this issue out into the open, make it a water cooler topic, and bring life and vitality back into the lives of millions of men and their partners.

> *I don't think I'm all that unusual—most women who notice something "off" in their romantic lives tend to blame themselves. There's so much guilt! I see women getting wrapped up in it all the time. The women I know definitely think of it as a personal rejection, plain and simple. It's not, but that's how they see it. I was so glad Sloan was able to get past it! It was like an old friend coming back again.*

If you haven't seen that "old friend" for awhile, and you miss him, then maybe the counsel in this book will help you to get reacquainted once more. It's never too late!

CHAPTER TWO

It's OK to Laugh

We might as well get them out of the way.

The jokes, I mean. Jokes about urologists. Jokes about sexual dysfunction. Jokes about anything related to male vitality, performance, or testicles. I've pretty much heard them all—many of them from one of the other seven urologists in my practice in Amarillo, Texas. Yes, they tell them, too. And as I'm one of the younger guys on staff, they love to direct many of them at me.

I like to stay in shape—this year for my 40th Birthday gift to myself I completed my first Ironman Triathlon—and my medical partners love to make fun of me for that. They all know how much I like to work out and watch my diet and stay away from junk food, and they laugh at me for it, in a good-natured kind of way. One day they pointed to a fellow with a bit of a potbelly and said to me, laughing, "See, in a couple of years, you're going to look just like him over there."

So you can probably imagine why I didn't tell them, until very recently, about my own experience with low testosterone. I knew the jokes would fly, and I wanted to avoid it as long as I could. But a few weeks ago, I decided to tell my laugh-loving colleagues about writing this book. And of course, I had to tell them, "I'm not only a doctor, I'm also a patient."

I had a pretty good idea how they'd react.

I finally made the announcement at the end of a recent monthly meeting. I cleared my throat and said, "Guys, I want you to know that I'm going to be writing a book about low testosterone. You all know I've been treating a growing number of men for it. But I'm pretty sure you didn't know that I started testosterone replacement therapy myself right about the time I joined you, five years ago."

It didn't take long. Sure enough, the jokes quickly began to fill the air. I don't remember the specific gags they told, but I'm sure they sounded a lot like the following (at least, the ones I can print):

"Hey Sloan, a ninety-year-old man went to his doctor for a checkup. 'You're in remarkable shape for a man your age,' said the doctor. 'I know it,' replied the old gentleman. 'I really have only one complaint—my sex drive is too high. Got anything you can do for that, Doc?' The doctor's mouth dropped open. 'Your *what*?' he gasped. 'My sex drive,' repeated the old man. 'It's too high, and I'd like to have you lower it, if you can.' 'Lower it?' cried the doctor. 'Just what do you consider "high"?' 'These days it seems like it's all in my head, Doc,' answered the elderly man, 'and I'd like to have you lower it a couple of feet if you can.'"

"Hey Sloan, what's the difference between your first honeymoon and your second? The first: Niagara; the second: Viagra."

"Hey Sloan, do you know why it takes one million sperm cells to fertilize one egg? They won't stop to ask for directions."

It went on like that for some time. And on. And on. Eventually I said, "Why do you guys think I waited five years to tell you about this? That is why, right there."

But of course, I laughed too. Because it *was* funny.

The Laughter Cycle

Guys, especially, seem to have a difficult time discussing subjects related to sex without making jokes about it. I don't claim to know why this might be, and anyway, it really doesn't matter much for the purposes of this book. I do think it's important to understand, however, that most guys *will* make jokes about the serious issues related to low testosterone . . . even if underneath all the joking, they have some serious questions.

Questions that go to the heart of what it means to be a man.

One of the most vivacious people I know on the planet is a very close family friend and the godfather to one of our sons. Not long ago my boys and I visited his ranch with a couple of other father/son groups. Whenever guys get together, of course, the topic of sex is bound to come up eventually. And almost always, soon afterward, the jokes and laughter kick into high gear. It was no different here.

At one point in our group conversation, however, I started telling my own story. I spoke about who can be affected by low testosterone and what it can do to a man's experience of life. Suddenly, every guy within earshot stopped all the banter, grew very quiet, and started listening intently. The dynamic fascinated me. And then, slowly at first, various guys started asking, "Um, could you tell me more about this? What are the symptoms? How . . .?"

I've learned through experience that the jokes and the jesting and the laughter can help guys to get ready to talk about more serious matters. All the chuckling and snickering can actually function as a doorway through which men can approach life-changing topics. That's very valuable—but I don't think that's the end of it. In fact, the purpose of discussing these serious matters is not merely to get serious; much more, it's so they can get back to the place in life where their experience can become enjoyable and interesting and compelling and fulfilling and satisfying and purposeful and *fun* once more.

Notice the important cycle here. Joking around enables us as men to discuss serious matters, which can give us the tools to recover our health and vitality, which in turn can bring a deeper laughter and even joy back into our lives. If you want a flow chart, think of it like this:

Joking around, serious discussion, deep joy, vitality, and renewed focus

And I don't need a study to tell me so, because my own recent experience reminds me that it is so.

From Black & White to Color

Before we begin with the more "clinical" part of this book, it might help for you to gain a greater acquaintance with Susan and I and our mutual history. Although the details of our story certainly differ from the particulars of others, it seems to me as though the general narrative thread looks, in many cases, quite similar. So don't be surprised if you see some of your own story in ours.

In essence, our story moves from color to black & white and then back again to color. Or from happy to drab and then a return to joy. Or from energetic to listless to energetic again … take your pick. We've seen the same basic trajectory over and over again. And since Susan has in many ways thought about it more deeply than I have, I think she should tell our story.

In 1990 I walked into a fraternity party at the University of Texas with my boyfriend at the time. Sloan was standing right by the door, and it was as though I saw little arrows pointing directly to him. I just knew. And he knew, too, even as a sophomore. We knew we were meant for each other. It was just a matter of time; there was no question about it. I know a lot of people don't have that sense of certainty, but I consider it a gift. I've never taken it for granted.

We got married in June right after I graduated in May. Even at our wedding, we looked around and thought, We are so blessed- our future is bright.

Originally Sloan thought he would go into business, but in college he figured out that wasn't for him. Next he tried to get into veterinary school, but those doors closed. We knew as one door is shut, another would open. Sloan had decided to become a doctor. He was accepted into the medical school at the University of Texas at Galveston, and despite all the long hours and constant demands to study, we had a blast. We dug in together. All tests took place on the first day of the school week; students called it "Black Monday." But after that it was fun, fun, fun, and then we'd work hard again. Half of the time when I talk about those days, people think I attended medical school along with Sloan, because I tend to say, "we." "We" took an anatomy class. We've always worked as a team.

At Galveston, the chief resident in urology was a family friend who earlier had urged Sloan to think about medicine as a career. Now he urged Sloan to consider urology as a specialty. We will always be grateful to Jeff for the mentor he is to Sloan. On Sloan's first day on campus, Jeff introduced him to the chairman of urology at UTMB, and after that Sloan sat in on some sessions with students and residents. The chairman sometimes asked him questions that more senior med students weren't getting. So urology seemed like a good and natural choice.

School was both fun and challenging. We both got into exercise and both loved to swim. A lot of "medical marriages" don't make it, but Galveston didn't seem difficult in that sense for either of us. We made life-long friends there and we all supported each other. During his first year of school, we talked so much about his class cadaver that he ruined my appetite every evening. I put up with that for one whole semester. So finally I decided to give him a self-portrait of my skull. Merry Christmas! We just had a lot of fun.

Sloan tends to have a very even personality, so I never noticed if he seemed to be in a good or a bad mood. I say he was "a forty-year-old at age twenty." He was my rock, and very consistent. During his emergency room rotations, for example, people would tell me that even when trauma patients arrived, his tone of voice never changed. He is very confident and calm in a crisis. He once saved the life of our next-door neighbor's two-year-old son. When the boy stopped breathing and started turning blue, his dad immediately brought his son over to Sloan. No change, he stays calm, no hysteria. He saved the boy's life without pomp or circumstance. For the first ten years of our marriage, Sloan was a very happy, laid back, consistent husband and father.

Things seemed to change after we arrived in Shreveport, Louisiana, for his residency in urologic surgery. Everything quickly grew more intense. I just kept thinking, OK, it's different. We've turned the heat up a little bit. And that's fine. After all, we had more or less asked God to do that very thing. We believed we had the opportunity to stay in Galveston, where it would have been safe and comfortable—but we thought it also would not be the same challenge for us that we knew we'd find at Shreveport. We'd asked for the heat to get turned up, so I figured we just had to take it.

Sloan was gone a lot during our years there, so I spent a lot of time with our two boys, watching football. We'd get in our jerseys and watch Game Day on ESPN and cheer on college football, because I wanted them to be able to do "guy stuff." We had a good time, but I couldn't help but notice that some things were changing with Sloan. I don't know exactly how to describe it; I found the symptoms very easy to explain away. We'd already had to work hard, and while this was certainly harder, something was slowly changing, just enough to notice. Sloan was becoming … different.

He became more isolated and showed little interest in people, which was always a core trait of his. He became very solitary and quiet and stoic—non-emotional, almost flatlined. Not angry, not mean, not sad. He remained loving and sweet, but in a very stoic way. Mentally, he was never able to focus on his medical texts more than fifty minutes at a time. And he couldn't study except in the morning, thirty to forty minutes, max. He simply couldn't concentrate more than that.

But honestly, none of those changes bothered me a lot until they started affecting our sex life. I didn't expect Sloan to have a huge, wonderful blast of an experience during residency. I knew going into it that I would have to carry more of the yoke. I was prepared for that. And I never worried about him having an affair, even though affairs were happening all around us. People were cheating on their spouses up at the hospital and allowed the flirting to get way out of control. When you're up there at all hours of the night and not at home with your family, a natural disconnect tends to happen. But spiritually and emotionally, Sloan always made me feel like the most beautiful girl in the room, even in his stoic period. So that wasn't it. He just didn't feel like talking—at all. And it wasn't mainly his mood change that I noticed, but rather the sexual side of our marriage. And even then, although his lack of interest bothered me, it didn't alarm me until I told him I'd like to have another child, and he responded with no desire for sex at all.

That mortified me.

At that point, I started to really doubt myself. Was I the problem? I went through the list of possible reasons for his rejection and kept asking myself, "What's wrong with me? What's wrong with me?" After a long time, finally I said to myself, "Uh-uh. I'm not the problem. He is." That's I when I confronted him with it, and that's when he got checked.

When the diagnosis came back, in one sense it was a big relief to know that Sloan's lack of sexual desire stemmed from a very low testosterone level; but to be honest, it wasn't the answer I wanted. What answer did I want? I don't know. I had no real expectations that I was aware of. Sloan and I talk a lot about how things in life can disappoint you really fast if you have particular expectations. I had none.

Still, it bothered me psychologically that he had to take an "injection" to feel sexual desire for me. I found it offensive, frankly. I remember thinking, *Why would he need to take a shot to be attracted to me? I look good. I look cute. I'm fun to be around.* I never expressed that opinion, so far as I remember, but I always felt more than a little skeptical about the whole thing. I thought, *I've never heard of this. Even **you** haven't really heard of this. Where's this coming from?* In my book, it seemed to be coming out of left field, like some kind of placebo effect. I thought, *Well, if it makes him feel better, great.* But at first, it deeply offended me.

I think that's a common reaction among many women, one that probably gets more common as we age. Wives think, *Am I not pretty? Am I no longer attractive?* A lot of women I know don't like the idea that their man has to take a pill in order to be "normal." It crushes your confidence and spirit- as it did mine.

I had to learn that men who suffer from low testosterone need medical help, every bit as much as if they had suffered a broken leg or a bloody injury in a car accident. These days Sloan likes to go mountain biking with guys a decade or more younger than he is—not something I'm always thrilled about—and if he were to get into a bad accident, God forbid, I wouldn't stop him from going to the emergency room because I thought he should just snap out of it. Wounds need to be sewn up; breaks need casts. And many men with low testosterone can regain their mojo with a little medical help. It's really that simple.

Today, Sloan is himself again—not younger, but back in color. For the longest time, it seemed like he was in black & white. The color had drained out of every pore in his body and he walked and talked and interacted only in shades of gray. Shortly after he started the therapy, however, he became confident and happy once more. The color returned to our lives! Today we're full partners again, having a lot of fun. Of course, there are days when he loses his patience and gets frustrated; but most of the time, he's laughing and enjoying life. He was always diligent and dutiful, even in his Stoic days, but now once more there's full engagement and a vibrant connection. I don't know how to say it any better: Sloan is back in color!

And boy, do I love that.

Go Ahead and Laugh

To succeed in urology, I believe you must have a robust sense of humor. I mean, let's be honest: Think about what we're dealing with, day after day. Urology is a very hands-on practice, and some of the things we have to put our hands on simply cry out for laughter.

During what was probably the last month of my residency, I had an unforgettable experience with a crack-up of a nurse. Now, urology nurses tend to be real characters, because to do what they have to do, it's almost a requirement. They just *have* to laugh. They like to tell jokes, too, but most of those will never appear in a book like this one.

I'll never forget this particular nurse; she always made me laugh. One day we had to treat a psychotic inmate who suffered from priapism (if you don't know what that is, I'll let you look it up). So we had him in the treatment room, and I had to put some needles into his body to drain off some blood, and then squeeze the affected portion of his body to force the blood out and get things back to normal.

I looked at the nurse and deadpanned, "And this is my job. *Really?*" She almost died laughing. (And I'm glad the psychotic inmate either had a sense of humor, or had checked out for a while.)

You know, it really is OK to laugh. Sometimes, in fact, it's almost required.

In the rest of this book I don't promise a lot of laughs, but I will do my best to give you some information, counsel, suggestions, and motivation to respond effectively and successfully to one of the most significant but least-publicized health challenges facing men today. **I consider a healthy testosterone level to be the secret to a man's mental, physical and sexual wellness.** If you're a man who may need a little help in this area, or if you love a man who you think may need such help, then I believe I can point you in the right direction. There's no reason to keep living in black & white when you can enjoy full color!

If you haven't laughed in a while—really *laughed*—then it's high time you got reacquainted with the experience. Hey, I'm a urologist, and I know what I'm talking about. Take it from me.

Please.

CHAPTER THREE

The Signs and Symptoms of Low T

"Jeff" visited me one afternoon at the clinic, mostly under protest. He didn't really see the point, he said; at least he was upfront about that. He had made the appointment, frankly, only after his wife, "Kelly," had put her foot down. She'd been after him for some time to get a checkup—she'd noticed some changes that troubled her—and none of her suggestions or recommendations had moved Jeff to call the doctor. So finally one day Kelly said, "That's enough. Either you make the appointment, or I will."

Jeff made the appointment.

And now here he sat, in my office physically, despite protesting in spirit. Jeff disinterestedly listed a few of the reasons for his wife's concern, while at the same time making it clear he thought all of his "symptoms" merely reflected his age. After all, he smirked, he wasn't a twenty-year-old anymore. These things just happen.

We briefly discussed the possible causes for his symptoms, he took a blood test, and then we scheduled a follow-up appointment. By the end of our first visit, Jeff clearly thought the appointment had been a waste of his time and money. But willingly went through it if it would help to silence Kelly.

A couple of weeks later, Jeff returned to my office, as promised. His attitude hadn't changed much. He told me again that he came because he didn't see any way out of it. He fully expected to find out that he'd been right all along.

So when I told him that his tests revealed he had about a third of the testosterone levels expected of a man his age (mid-30s), and that the low numbers very likely had led directly to the symptoms that had so concerned his wife, suddenly I had his full attention. His facial expression instantly turned from bored to shocked . . . and then, maybe more than a little alarmed. I let the news sink in a bit, and then for the first time, we had a serious discussion about the possible benefits of testosterone replacement therapy.

Today, both Jeff and Kelly are *much* happier campers.

Red Flags, or At Least Orange Ones

The FDA reports that at least 15 million men in America suffer from Low Testosterone. Yet only about 5 percent of them are ever diagnosed and treated, which means 95 percent are either misdiagnosed or never diagnosed at all. This means Low Testosterone may be one of the most overlooked and under-diagnosed of all medical conditions, partly because many men who suffer from it don't recognize the symptoms—in part, because the symptoms start showing up gradually, in most cases making their appearance over years or decades rather than weeks or months. But it's also because, like Jeff, many men dismiss the symptoms as "part of aging." For very similar reasons, some medical professionals don't even consider checking a patient for Low T, even though he may suffer from some or more of its most common symptoms.

So how can you know if you, or the man in your life, should get examined and tested for Low T? Consider a few of the telltale signs and symptoms of Low T. Please keep in mind that the presence of any of these is no proof of Low T—only tests performed by a physician can reveal that—but they may well signal a problem.

Three basic categories of symptoms signal Low Testosterone: the sexual, the physical, and the mental/emotional. Let's briefly consider the symptoms associated with each.

Sexual Symptoms

When most people think of the term "Low Testosterone," their minds probably go first to the effects the condition can have on a man's sex life. There is no doubt that men who suffer from Low T often realize something has gone wrong when they stop desiring sex (or when they desire it much less than before) or when they are unable to "perform" as well as they'd like.

Loss of Sexual Desire (Low Libido)

Probably the best-known and most discussed sexual problem is erectile dysfunction (ED), the inability to achieve and maintain an erection sufficient for sexual intercourse (we have waves of television and radio commercials to thank for that!). We'll get to ED soon, but first let's take a look at another Low T-related sexual issue: the loss of libido.

Simply put, the libido is the desire for sex, also known as the sex drive or sex hunger. A male's libido is largely driven by his testosterone level, so it is only natural that a man's desire for sex will level off or decrease as he ages. It's no secret that a typical man in his mid-40s won't have nearly as an intense sex drive as he did in his late teens and early 20s. Many of us would probably argue that this is, in many ways, a good thing!

But the natural decrease in testosterone level in most men shouldn't cause a complete (or almost complete) loss of desire for sex. Most males with normal, healthy testosterone levels will still have the "desire," even if it doesn't feel as all-consuming as it did in their younger years. But when the condition called Low T enters the picture, that desire for sex can be one of the first casualties.

This change can feel very traumatic, both for the man and for his partner. A healthy, intimate relationship is one of the most important keys to a happy marriage. For an otherwise healthy man, losing his desire for sex can feel worse than losing a lifelong friend. His libido is part of what makes him male, and when it starts to disappear, he begins to wonder what's wrong with him … and if it can be fixed. He feels, frankly, like less of a man.

And of course, the woman in the relationship wonders the same thing—*about herself.* Her mind wanders toward emotionally wrenching questions like:

- *Am I no longer attractive to him?*
- *Have I put on too much weight?*
- *Have I done or said something to turn him off?*
- *Is there another woman … or man?*

If you remember, my own experience with Low T eventually prompted my own wife, Susan, to ask many of these very questions. It took her some time, constantly running these self-accusatory questions through her mind, before she finally concluded (correctly!) that the problem didn't lie with her, but with me.

Susan and I went through the same kinds of struggles that so many couples do when the man in the relationship suffers from Low Testosterone, and doesn't know it. In our case, it wasn't that I had stopped loving my wife, and it certainly wasn't that I wanted someone else. I simply thought of myself as a largely contented—if overly busy— man trying to make his mark on the world. I doubted I had time to think about much else.

I had no clue I had a medical condition that needed prompt attention.

Erectile Dysfunction (ED)

You don't have to watch a lot of television, listen to a lot of radio, or read a lot of magazines to know that drugs treating erectile dysfunction have become big business in the United States. Prescription medications such as sildenafil (Viagra), vardenafil (Levitra) and tadalafil (Cialis) all have become household names in the past few decades; and depending on the patient's circumstances, all of them can be effective.

ED and the decrease of libido do not necessarily go hand-in-hand. Some patients report that although they still feel the desire, they simply no longer have the ability to do anything about it. On the other hand, some patients report that they can achieve strong erections, but just don't have much interest in sex anymore.

Like other common symptoms of Low T, erectile dysfunction often points to other health issues, as well—some of which can be extremely serious. Some of the conditions associated with ED are high blood pressure, high cholesterol, heart disease, and diabetes. ED can also be caused by fatigue, stress, physical injuries, smoking, and excessive alcohol consumption.

Like the loss of libido, ED is very often one of the symptoms of Low T. It is also one of the symptoms that grows worse over time as a man ages and his testosterone level drops. Most men go from experiencing spontaneous erections (especially in their teens and 20s) to needing more and more stimulation to become erect. Many men with Low T seem barely able to achieve enough of an erection for sex.

Problems with Climax/Sensation

Many men with Low T have trouble reaching climax during sex. This is sometimes because of decreased sensitivity in the penis, yet another symptom of Low T. While most men with adequate levels of testosterone have no difficulty reaching climax in a short amount of time, men with Low T sometimes "take forever" to reach orgasm—and some even "fake it" when they grow tired of the effort. Men with Low T also frequently report the loss of "morning erections"; men with normal levels of testosterone often have such erections, because their testosterone levels are at their highest in the early morning.

Mental/Emotional Symptoms

Several mental/emotional symptoms can point to a problem with Low Testosterone. Very often, these kinds of symptoms appear obvious to a man's partner, or even to anyone who spends a lot of time around him. These symptoms include:

- Fatigue
- Poor Concentration/Trouble Thinking
- Lack of Energy/Initiative
- Depression
- Moodiness/Irritability

To this day, my wife remembers how, during my residency, I began to demonstrate some of the mental symptoms associated with Low T. I had a very difficult time concentrating on anything for an extended period of time—which is a big problem for a young medical student going through residency! The longest I could focus on any one task was thirty to forty minutes—fifty on a really good day.

I also had a hard time remembering things—again, not a good situation for a medical student in residency. I can't honestly say good memory has ever been a strength of mine, but during that period I had extreme difficulty remembering names or many of the things I had just read and studied. I had to read my textbooks over and over in order to file away the important data in my brain.

Finally, I lost some interest in many of the most important things in life, including my family and my friendships. I wasn't what most people would think of as moody or irritable, but my temperament had changed. I remember how everything seemed "gray" to me. I didn't enjoy the things that before I had found delightful, and I disengaged from or gave up involvement with the people or things I had highly valued. As Susan remembers it, I didn't laugh or smile much. I withdrew and became very solitary (something not in my nature), quiet, and stoic.

In short, I just wasn't myself—and my wife could see it, even if I couldn't.

One reason it can be so difficult to recognize the mental/emotional symptoms of Low T is that so many factors can cause a man to feel fatigued, moody, depressed, and irritable. I was in the middle of my residency, and married with two small children. With everything I had going on, it would have been a miracle if I *hadn't* gone through at least some of those emotions, at least some of the time. Like most men, I was too busy in my career to notice subtle changes. I attributed things to "aging"—and lowered my standards.

That is why it is very important to recognize a broad range of the symptoms of Low T. That way, you can be one step ahead in discovering if the problem really is Low T and not simple fatigue, depression, or another stress-related emotion.

Non-Sexual Physical Symptoms

As a man ages, it's perfectly normal for him to see changes in his physique. The muscle mass he saw building in his 20s and early 30s declines and he starts losing the ability to perform athletically the way he once did. He can't run as fast, lift as much, or jump as high.

If you need a quick illustration of this point, just pay close attention to the ages of the athletes competing in the summer or winter Olympics, or in professional sports leagues. Chances are, most of them are under 30, and very few of them are over 35.

Those of us in our late 30s or early 40s (and even beyond) who once competed in athletics or who spent a great amount of time exercising and "staying in shape" know how discouraging it can be to lose the physical abilities we once had. But there is no reason a healthy man can't continue to make exercise and fitness a part of his life, well past his 40s and 50s. He shouldn't expect to have the same results he did in his 20s, but that's just a part of life.

Low Testosterone, however, can exacerbate the decline and keep a man from enjoying full health throughout his life span.

Decrease in Muscle Mass/Tone

One of the effects of testosterone in a young man's body is the development of larger and stronger muscles. As a man ages and as his testosterone level drops, some decline in his muscle mass and tone also will occur. But when a man notices *big* losses in his muscle mass and tone—in other words, his muscles seem small and not as defined—then it may be that he suffers from Low T and needs to see his doctor. Nothing is more frustrating than putting in the time at the gym, but not seeing the results.

Decrease in Strength/Stamina & Athletic Performance

When muscle mass and tone decrease, declines in strength, stamina, and athletic performance usually follow close behind. Any man over the age of 35 or 40—unless he's living in the past—knows he can't lift as much, run as fast, and jump as high as he once could. That's natural, but again, when a man loses much of his strength, stamina, and athletic ability over a relatively short time, or if the losses are more extreme than might be expected for his age, it may be because he has Low T.

Unexplained Weight Gain

Another common symptom of Low T is weight gain—especially around the mid-section. As I'll explain later, many men who just can't seem to lose the "love handles"—and who have been diagnosed with Low T— find that they *can* lose the extra weight once they receive treatment for their condition.

So…What's *Really* Wrong with Him?

If you see the symptoms outlined above in yourself, or if you see them in the man you love, please don't ignore them. They could point to Low T, or other serious health conditions, and they likely will not improve without treatment.

While any of us can recognize most of the signs and symptoms of Low T, only a doctor can tell if that is the core problem, or if the symptoms signal some other health problem. If your doctor performs the necessary blood tests and identifies the problem as Low T, then the time has come to talk to him or her about treatments that can bring that testosterone level back to normal—and keep it there.

Low T … Or Something Else?

Before I conclude this chapter, I think it's important to understand that as a man ages, his testosterone levels *will* decline. That's just as natural (though not usually as noticeable) as the process of puberty he endured during adolescence. And as a man's testosterone level declines, he will go through several physical changes. His sex drive and his body shape and tone will change. The main question is whether the man maintains a high enough level of testosterone to keep the changes from being too drastic and to keep him healthy and happy.

The testosterone levels of the typical human male spike between the ages of 14 and 20. Testosterone levels tend to level off during the 20s and 30s, but after the age of 40, they begin to decline steadily—at an average rate of 1 to 2 percent per year. By middle age, almost all men will have undergone a fairly substantial decline in their testosterone levels.

Several conditions can cause Low T—certain chronic diseases, trauma/injury to the testicles, rare chromosomal abnormalities, pituitary tumors or other problems, and drug and alcohol abuse. But in my experience, in the *overwhelming* majority of cases—I'd say higher than 90 percent—Low T is caused by the simple fact that the testicles aren't producing it like they used to, simply because the man is aging and his body starts producing less testosterone. This is sometimes called "andropause."

I'd like to re-emphasize, too, that the symptoms associated with Low T also could be associated with other physical issues. While some are relatively minor (the man might simply need more rest or more regular exercise), some are very serious, even life-threatening problems, such as heart disease or sleep apnea. *Only a medical professional can accurately diagnose whether you or the man you love has Low T*—or another serious condition that needs attention.

Two things are required for a valid diagnosis of Low T: results from taking a questionnaire designed to determine the presence of relevant symptoms (see the sidebar Teeple's Testosterone Test), and results from a physician-administered blood test. Together, these tests can determine beyond any doubt if the patient suffers from Low T.

And what does a physician or clinician look for when testing for Low T? Testosterone is considered low with a score of under 300, meaning less than 300 nanograms (a nanogram is the unit for measurement used in measuring various hormones in blood tests, including testosterone) of testosterone per deciliter of blood. A score of between 300 and 400 may or may not be low, depending on the symptoms of the patient. A score higher than 400 is usually considered normal—again, depending on the patient's clinical symptoms. "Free" testosterone levels provide yet another gauge, and a level below 12 pg/ml is also considered low. Bottom line—if either the Total T is low OR the Free T is low and a patient has symptoms, then the man may be a candidate for Testosterone Replacement Therapy.

Happy Camping to You

Jeff didn't want to see me about the symptoms his wife had been noticing in him, and I've discovered that he's not at all unusual. Most men would rather ignore the symptoms or chalk them up to their increasing years. Thank God for the concerned women in their lives!

Jeff and Kelly's story had a happy ending because Kelly insisted her husband get checked. Would they be happy campers right now if his Low T had gone undiagnosed, and more importantly, untreated? I'll let you ponder that one.

In the meanwhile, I hope that some happy camping is in your future, too, if it's not already in your present. I know I'm glad I've got someone to help me keep my sleeping bag warm.

Teeple's Testosterone Test

www.TeeplesTestosteroneTest.com
Testosterone—What it Is and What it Does

Testosterone is a naturally occurring—and very important—steroid hormone produced mostly in the testicles of the male, in the ovaries of the female, and in the adrenal glands of both sexes. Women's bodies produce and use testosterone, but at levels far lower than in men—around 1/10th that of the average male.

As you read that last paragraph, the word *steroid* may have jumped out at you. That's understandable, because over the past few decades that word has taken quite a beating, especially among those of us who enjoy watching "manly" spectator sports such as football, basketball, and baseball. Unfortunately, many, if not most, people today associate naturally occurring steroids with the performance-enhancing chemicals and compounds some athletes have taken in order to "gain an edge" on their competition. You need to know that the few athletes that do abuse steroids are using 10 to 100 times the normally prescribed doses of testosterone.

To understand how important testosterone and other naturally occurring steroids are for a man's health and well-being, we need to step away from that kind of thinking about the word *steroid*. In truth, our bodies produce and make use of several important steroid hormones—some of which are essential to life. For example, a lack of the steroid hormone cortisol, which is also produced in the adrenal glands, can threaten one's life. Other naturally occurring steroid hormones include estrogen (the primary female sex hormone), progesterone, and aldosterone.

The simplest way to describe hormones is by using the term "chemical messengers." A hormone essentially is a naturally-produced chemical released from a cell or gland that carries signals or messages to other parts of the body to tell the body do a certain thing. Testosterone is one of dozens of hormones in the human body, and each of them serves a specific purpose.

Testosterone is the primary male sex hormone, and it serves several purposes. Testosterone is the main engine for producing what are called secondary sex characteristics in males. Secondary sex characteristics are the non-reproductive features that distinguish the males and the females of a particular species. In the animal kingdom, most species have secondary sex characteristics. In human males, the secondary sex characteristics produced by testosterone include:

- Growth of body and facial hair, as well as the loss of scalp hair in some men
- Greater muscle and bone mass

- Enlargement of the larynx (Adam's apple)
- Deepening of the voice
- Greater muscle mass and strength
- Broadening of shoulders and chest

The effects of testosterone in a man's life are most obvious during puberty. During that time (in a young male's early teens, give or take a few years), a rush of new testosterone causes some profound and obvious bodily changes. A young man's muscles and bones begin to grow larger (a process that continues well into his 20s), his voice deepens, he begins growing hair in places that lacked hair before, and, of course, his sex drive begins to rev up.

Even after puberty, the man's body makes use of testosterone in several important ways. The hormone is crucial for the general health and well-being of a fully grown man. It plays a part in regulating a man's sex drive, his mood, his mental health, his aggressiveness (or initiative/energy), and his general feeling of well-being.

Without a proper amount of testosterone pulsing through his veins, a human male would never develop the larger muscles and bones, would never grow facial hair, wouldn't develop a deep voice, and wouldn't broaden in the shoulders and chest. He also would likely be more prone to moodiness, depression, fatigue, and other symptoms of Low T.

Simply put, testosterone is the hormone responsible for making a man, a man—but also for making him a happy, healthy man! And when you consider the many roles testosterone plays in helping make a human male a happy, healthy, balanced man, it only makes sense that a low supply of testosterone would have a negative impact on many parts of his life.

CHAPTER FOUR

Broaching the Subject

Ways to Approach Him if You Think He May Have Low T

Jake and Valerie Johnson[1] had a great relationship through most of their marriage. But as the years went by, Jake changed. He couldn't function sexually, on the rare occasions when he even tried. It got to the point where Viagra offered no help. Even trying things like putting a latch on the bedroom door—Valerie wondered if this shy, reserved man worried that the kids might hear them or, worse yet, walk into the bedroom during their lovemaking—had no effect.

At the same time, Jake's mood also became more and more somber, to the point where he had every symptom of clinical depression. Nothing Valerie tried seemed to help. Even in those increasingly rare moments when Jake seemed interested in sexual intimacy, he couldn't achieve a hard enough erection for sexual intercourse. And even when he did get a firm erection, it didn't last.

Valerie and Jake had reached the "empty nest" part of their family life. Their kids had grown up and had moved away, leaving

---

1   Not their real names.

just the two of them. They had come to a time of life that many men dream about: the "second honeymoon" period of their marriage. Valerie and Jake loved one another and would have loved to enjoy the newfound privacy for which they'd sacrificed over so many years. But their hopes went unrealized—simply because, like so many men who reach this life stage, Jake's desire for renewed passion and romance with his wife ran head-on into a steep drop in his testosterone levels.

Valerie felt the sexual frustration that a similar situation would cause anyone (she described it "like spinning around on a ceiling fan"), but even worse was the effect that Jake's lack of sexual function had on her self-esteem. Like many wives of sexually dysfunctional men, Valerie began to look inward and not at the possible physical causes of Jake's problem. ***Why does the man I love not want me?*** she wondered. And she couldn't stop wondering about it.

As a child, Valerie had endured terrible abuse; at one point, she had given up on the idea, not just of being married, but on men, period. So when the man she finally married, whom she had loved so deeply for so many years, either didn't seem interested in being intimate with her or couldn't perform on those rare occasions when the interest materialized, she felt devastated.

The self-doubt continued to grow, and so did the feeling that she somehow deserved what was happening. "I believed I was getting punished for something," she said. "I wondered if I had let God down."

To make matters worse, when she talked to Jake's doctor about the situation—that Jake seemed depressed and tired all the time and that he couldn't perform sexually—she felt completely ignored. Valerie remembers one doctor, an elderly man, who said, "Jake, you're working too hard at it! Slap her on the butt, and turn over and go to sleep." (Actually, Valerie remembers the doctor wasn't even *that* nice about it; but that's how she describes the hurtful incident today.)

The situation continued to deteriorate for several years, and Valerie grew ever more convinced that somehow she had caused the problem. Of course, she hadn't.

Finally, some fifteen years before I met the Johnsons, a short-lived glimmer of hope appeared. Another doctor listened as Valerie listed Jake's symptoms; finally he put Jake on the testosterone patch. Jake's moods started improving and his sexual performance increased, but when he stopped using the patch due to the rashes it caused, the symptoms returned—worse than ever, as Valerie recalls. Sex once a week turned into once every two weeks, then once a month, before it stopped altogether.

A Turning Point for Jake

Valerie consulted with me for several years before she decided the time had come to persuade Jake to see me, too. The two hadn't made love in more than a year, and she deeply missed the closeness of physical intimacy she had enjoyed with Jake.

As she saw it, if Jake didn't get some help, she had only two options: step outside her marriage for it (which she never would have considered), or live the rest of her life in a sexless, passionless marriage.

The turning point came when the couple went on a camping trip. Finally, Valerie summoned up the courage to ask Jake the question asked by so many wives of men with Low T: "Jake, do you just not find me appealing?"

Jake, a very reserved man who has a difficult time with such conversations ("a man of few words," Valerie says) summoned up the inner strength to confess, "Well, Valerie, I have a problem."

"Why didn't you tell me?" Valerie asked.

"Because it's embarrassing," he replied.

The tears welled up in Valerie's eyes as her mind began racing from one terrible possibility to another. Again, she summoned up the courage to ask the question to which she might not like the answer: "Well, what is your problem?"

Jake hesitated and then confessed, "I'm going to have to be circumcised."

About thirty-five years before, Jake had suffered an accident in which superheated water badly scalded him, leaving him with first-, second-, and third-degree burns over 80 percent of his body; the worst damage occurred below the waist. The scars had led to some discomfort during sex, especially since Jake had never been circumcised.

Circumcised? That's all? Valerie thought. "For gosh sakes," she said, "we could have had *that* taken care of years ago!"

Valerie didn't wait. She asked Jake if he felt ready to see a doctor, and he replied, "I might as well, because you're going to do something about it, anyway."

"That's right!" she declared. "I'm going to take care of you any way I can."

Valerie called my office and made an appointment. When Jake and Valerie arrived for their visit, I asked Jake to fill out a questionnaire. Valerie immediately took pen in hand and began asking Jake questions, writing down his answers one by one. When she finished filling out the questionnaire, I looked at the answers and mentally went through the checklist of his symptoms. Decreased sex drive? Yes. Decrease in sexual function, including erectile dysfunction? Yes. Lack of energy and constant fatigue? Yes and yes.

Jake didn't have all the hallmark symptoms of Low T (many men who suffer from the condition don't), but he responded "yes" enough times to justify a blood test. When the results came back positive for Low T, I put him on a prescription for Androgel. Jake began applying the gel every night, right after his shower.

The Androgel began helping Jake almost right away. He became more like himself as the testosterone kicked in, and his sex drive and ability to perform sexually returned. His recovery, however, did not proceed without having to overcome some problems early on in his treatment.

It shocked Valerie to see how Jake became very aggressive—a side-effect in some men as treatment begins. This formerly mild-mannered, passive man became aggressive in ways very unlike him. "I would say something to him and he would bite my head off," Valerie remembers. "But then I could see it starting to level out."

Once Jake's moods evened out, Valerie welcomed back the man she always had loved. He no longer seemed depressed and his self-esteem returned to a healthy level. She even noticed that he began losing weight, and complimented him on it. Today, the Johnsons have a happy marriage in which they again enjoy being with one another—in every way.

Remember how Viagra couldn't help the Johnsons' sex life? Now they don't even need it.

Valerie's Approach

Valerie faced the same situation that countless women married to testosterone-deficient men have to deal with: how to bring up the possibility that his symptoms may point to the medical condition called Low T. It's not as simple as you might think; when many men hear the words, "Honey, I think you need to get your testosterone checked," what they hear is, "Baby, let's get you to the doctor so we can find out if you actually *are* a man."

The last thing Valerie wanted to do was make a bad situation worse by saying something her husband could badly misconstrue. For many years—the years in which Jake couldn't perform sexually—Valerie attempted to prod her husband toward an appointment with his doctor by pointing out that she knew of members of her family who had remained sexually active into their seventies and even eighties. Jake never bought the story, so he never made that initial visit to the doctor to get checked out.

With Plan A in ruins, what could Valerie do? She couldn't help but notice that Jake's mood and self-esteem had plummeted; so even though she suspected that at least part of his problem might be low testosterone, she knew she couldn't just blurt out, "Hey, you need to get your testosterone levels checked!" Such an approach, she knew, would have depleted whatever self-esteem he had left.

"One of a woman's privileges and responsibilities as a wife is to build up her husband's self-esteem," she said, "not tear it down—even inadvertently."

Valerie knew she would have to take a kinder, gentler approach. So she approached the necessary conversation with an attitude of equality. She pointed out that, as they age, many women need estrogen treatments in order to retain their sex drive. And if she needed estrogen treatment herself, she had at least a basic idea of what Jake might be going through and how he felt about it.

"If I needed estrogen, then men might need something, too, because God made us in a similar way," she said. She figured she would let Jake's doctor tell him how his depression, fatigue, and loss of sexual function could be related to low testosterone levels. That way, she said, she could avoid the charge of taking a "know-it-all" attitude.

Valerie suggests that one of the most important things a woman can do for her partner is to continually support him and affirm him— doubly important as he seeks diagnosis and possible treatment for Low T. Valerie's advice: Remind him that he's still all man, and make him *feel* like a man—the man you love. That includes speaking loving words, both to him and to others, that communicate just how much you respect him, love him, and feel good to be with him. And, of course, this includes letting him know that you love his body and want to be with him sexually.

"Brag on them and tell them they're sexy," she said. "I don't care if they're eighty years old or twenty, men like to hear that as much as women do."

Who Knows Him Better?

In my practice, I've heard from and worked with many women who have faced the same sort of situation that bedeviled Valerie. She knew and loved her man more than she could put into words, and she wanted the very best for him, and for their marriage. But she also found out—the hard way—that many men simply don't want to hear that their bodies may not be producing enough testosterone to keep them healthy mentally and physically.

But if *anyone* could understand that something had gone physically wrong with Jake, that someone was Valerie. They had lived together for decades as a happily married couple; they knew one another better than anyone else, and so when things started going downhill for Jake, Valerie knew they had to do something.

What about you? If you're reading this book, then it may be that you've recognized that your mate has lost a little something over the years—his "mojo," as many might put it. So how can you approach your man when you suspect he may be suffering from Low T?

First, keep in mind that no one knows your man better than you do. You know his personality quirks, his temperament, what makes him happy, sad, angry, or excited, and you certainly know what turns him on sexually. In other words, you know what makes him, him! And when some or all of those things start to change, you notice it. In fact, many times these things are impossible to miss. Since you know him so well, therefore, doesn't it just make sense that you would be the one to encourage, nudge, or even push him toward identifying the problem, whether it's Low T or another physical or mental/emotional problem that needs attention?

This book won't teach you everything there is to know about testosterone. Frankly, a lot of what the medical community knows (or doesn't know) about how testosterone affects a man wouldn't help you much as you consider what to do when you suspect your man may suffer from Low T. Still, by now you should know enough to be able to look at your mate and evaluate how he's been feeling and acting, and weigh what you see against what you now know are the telltale symptoms of Low T. Do whatever you must do in order to help and encourage him to take a course of action that will lead him back to full health. Everybody needs a little help, now and again.

Now the big question: What *can* you do?

I've dedicated the rest of this chapter to showing you how to best approach your man if you suspect he may suffer from Low T. As with most medical or emotional/mental problems, this subject can be difficult to broach. It becomes all the more difficult, however, because of the mentality of most men when it comes to manhood in general and testosterone in particular.

So, a quick note before we move on: Please remember that your thinking and his are likely to differ substantially on this subject. Just bringing up your suspicion that he might suffer from Low T—let's say, in the same way you would if you thought he might be suffering from a bad case of the flu—will not likely produce the results you'd hoped for. Talking to your man about Low T probably will require every bit of tact and diplomacy you can muster.

Also, I didn't write this chapter as if it were a quick "by the numbers" set of instructions for how to talk to your mate about Low T. Consider what follows simply as some tidbits of wisdom gleaned from experience, both as a Low T patient myself and from having treated and counseled scores of Low T sufferers as a medical professional.

Educate Yourself

You probably don't have a mere passing interest in Low T. No doubt you've reached this point in the book because you've noticed certain troubling changes in your man and you know something's not right. And perhaps you've begun to suspect that this something just might be Low T.

Valerie emphasized the importance of informing herself before attempting to talk to her husband about Low T. She spoke of relatives and other acquaintances whose marriages fell apart due to the ravaging effects of Low T. Obtaining some readily available information on Low T, she believes, could save many otherwise troubled marriages.

I've found this to be especially important for wives of younger men—men in their 20s to 40s—who suffer or may suffer from Low T. A lot of these women haven't yet reached the point in the aging process where their bodies have started to produce less estrogen, so they have a difficult time relating to their husbands' problem. They sense that something has gone wrong, but they have no clue as to what it might be.

By now, you should have a basic knowledge of what testosterone is, what it does, and what can happen when a man's body stops producing enough of it. But you still might have some questions. If so, I've included a "Low T Q & A Appendix" at the end of this book that might more directly answer some of your questions. If after reading this book you still want to know more about the topic, you might look into some other resources.

First, read about the subject from as many sources as possible, whether books or magazines or on the Internet.

Second, once you've finished reading, write down your questions, especially those that relate directly to you and your partner. Keep these in a notebook or journal, or in another place where they won't get lost and can be retrieved easily.

Finally, make an appointment with a medical professional who specializes in Low T and other men's health issues. Come to your visit with your list of questions, and don't be afraid to explore all the areas that concern you.

Once you get your answers, it's time to ask more questions—but this time, of your mate.

Start With the Easy Ones and Move Up

Read though the following exchanges between a long-married husband and wife, and then ask yourself how they compare:

Exchange No. 1

> She: "Honey, I've noticed lately that you seem tired all the time, and that you don't seem to have much energy for anything. You seem grumpy and moody, and sometimes it's even hard for me to know how to talk to you. Lately you've been spending a lot more time by yourself, and when you're alone, you aren't doing anything but sitting around watching TV or sleeping. We haven't had sex in what seems like forever, and I wonder if you even *want* to be with me physically anymore. And something else—you're starting to put on some weight."

> He: "Well, maybe I've just been working too hard. I do feel tired a lot, so maybe it's time for a vacation or something. As for the weight, maybe I just need to hit the gym a little more often."

> She: "Dear, I think it might be more than that. I think you might have a problem I've been reading about lately: Low Testosterone. Let's make an appointment to talk to your doctor about it."

> He: "What? Are you *kidding* me? Why are you even reading about that stuff? There's nothing wrong with me. I'm fine! I just need some rest. Let's just drop it, OK?"

Exchange No. 2

> She: "Sweetheart, how have you been feeling lately? Have you been feeling a little tired or lethargic? I wonder if you have you been feeling physically weaker than you

used to. I'd sure like it if we made love more often, like we used to. I really enjoy being with you in that way."

He: "Now that you mention it, I *have* felt a little down lately. Yeah, I'm tired a lot and I don't have much energy. And I *do* feel a little weaker than usual lately. I didn't think you'd noticed. Maybe I should talk to our doctor about it."

She: "Well, isn't it nearly time for your yearly physical? Maybe we should talk to your doctor about how you've been feeling. Let's see if he might have some idea of how we can get you back to where you were before. And I wonder if maybe we should ask him to check out your testosterone levels? I hear that's a very common condition for a lot of men. It's also not that difficult to fix."

He: "Well … OK. So long as I'm getting poked and prodded anyway, I guess there's no harm in asking about *that*. I doubt that's the problem, though. But I guess we could ask the doc about it—you know, so long as we're already there."

The most obvious difference in the two verbal exchanges is the response from the man. In exchange No. 1, the man immediately put up his defenses when he heard the phrase, "low testosterone." The woman, though certainly she didn't mean for it to come out that way, unfortunately brought up the subject in what he perceived as an accusatory way. She unwittingly phrased it in a way that he heard as "You have a problem, bud!"

In the second exchange, the woman more or less led her man into a willingness to get his testosterone level checked *during his next physical*. She did so by asking questions, not by making observations about things he may or may not have noticed.

Ladies, you should know that when many of us men hear the phrase "low testosterone," we react much like we do when we hear the word "castration." Frankly, it makes us want to corkscrew ourselves into our chairs! That's why it's so important to start most conversations about the possibility of Low T with some of the same general questions the woman asked in Exchange No. 2.

Remember, you know your man better than anyone else knows him. Maybe the more direct approach—the one highlighted in Exchange No. 1—will yield the desired result. But I'd be willing to bet that, in the majority of cases, the "kinder, gentler" approach illustrated in Exchange No. 2 will work better.

If you have noticed that your mate is no longer interested in sex (or that his interest has waned more than you think it should have), that he seems lethargic or depressed or distant, and that his body is changing more rapidly than it should be, the time may have come to start asking the kinds of questions used in Exchange No. 2.

And consider something else as you begin asking your questions: Could it be that at least *some* of your partner's symptoms might result from other factors, such as stress at work? Most men know that pressure on the job can cause them to feel stressed, and stress can cause us to respond in ways that look a lot like one or another medical condition. So remember, even when the symptoms *look* very much like Low T (and that includes some of the sexual ones), they could simply result from stress.

Taking the Questions to Another Level

If your mate seems reluctant to answer the "kinder, gentler" questions, or if he resists the idea of seeing his doctor about the symptoms you've noticed (don't forget, many men are notorious for exactly that) you might need to move things up a notch or two.

Try asking him why he doesn't seem interested in you sexually the way he once was. Even if you've settled the "is it me?" questions for yourself, asking him these kinds of questions just might encourage him to ask why he doesn't seem interested in sex with you lately.

If you've asked all the questions suggested above and still he doesn't seem interested in seeing his doctor, you might have to move on to one of the shockers—just like my wife did. You've already read about how my not-a-wallflower wife, Susan, put herself through the litany of self-incriminating questions that so many women ask when they notice the symptoms of Low T in their man. She wondered if *she* could be the problem, if maybe *she* needed to make some changes. Once she felt satisfied that the problem was mine, she began asking *me* the questions.

Her final question about the nature of my sexuality finally shook me out of my lethargy and put me on a path toward wholeness and wellness. I thank God every day when I think of my wife's willingness to ask such a difficult question.

Questions like "are you having an affair?" might feel very difficult for you to ask because, quite honestly, you may fear his answers. *What if I ask him if he's having an affair, and the answer is "yes?" I couldn't bear to hear from his own mouth that he's been cheating on me! Worse yet, what if I ask him if he's cheating WITH ANOTHER MAN and the answer is "yes?"*

Your mate may not give you direct answers to some of these questions; but it's possible the questions themselves may get him thinking along a new track. Some of them may even shock him into doing some serious self-evaluation, as Susan's did with me. If that happens, you might find him willing at least to hear from his doctor.

I know it worked for me!

It's a Medical Condition, Not a Loss of Manhood

As we've seen, one big reason so many men have a difficult time even considering the possibility that they might suffer from Low T is the skewed thinking that goes like this: *If I have low T, then that means my body isn't working like a* real *man's body works. If I can't "get it up" and if I can't find it in me to work hard and be productive, then it's because I'm not a real man anymore.*

Trust me! I've heard this kind of thinking from *a lot* of men who suffer with Low T. Time after time, I've met men who had to overcome their reluctance even to bring up the subject. They fear that doing even that much amounts to acknowledging that they aren't the men they once were.

In many ways, this reluctance parallels how our society used to see mental illness. Not so long ago, our culture attributed mental illness to everything from weak character to low intellect to demonic influences. Today, we recognize mental illness as a medical condition, often a treatable one, just like cancer or heart disease.

No doubt you will get a lot further in encouraging your partner to find out if he suffers from Low T (and to seek treatment) if you remind him gently that Low T is a *treatable medical condition.* It's not a loss of manhood. Not even close!

Low T is not something to be ashamed of or embarrassed about, but rather something that affect millions of men without them even knowing it. Remember that fact as you seek to communicate your concerns with your mate, and as *a couple*, you begin the process of discovering whether your partner suffers from Low T.

CHAPTER FIVE

What Can We Do?

Treatment Options for Low T

In 1889, a 72-year old French physician named Charles-Edouard Brown-Sequard made news in medical circles when he stood before the Society de Biologie of Paris and announced that he had enjoyed some amazing personal results when he injected himself with a compound made out of the extract from the testicles of guinea pigs and dogs.

That same year, Brown-Sequard described the effects of his self-experimentation this way: *"a radical change took place in me. … I fully regained my old powers. … My limbs … showed a decided gain of strength. With regard to the facility of intellectual labour … a return to my previous ordinary condition became quite manifest during and after the first two or three days of my experiments."*

That all sounds reminiscent of what any man who suffers with Low T would want in a medication, doesn't it? Later on, however, examinations of Brown-Sequard's wonder extract showed little in the way of any kind of androgen, meaning the benefits he received from his injections were probably more of a placebo than anything else. In other words, the effects appeared to emanate all from his mind.

It might be a stretch to call Charles-Edouard Brown-Sequard the father of what is now called testosterone replacement therapy (TRT)—but then again, it might not. One thing is for sure: Brown-Sequard's studies and experiments, as strange and risky as they may seem today, led to increased interest among the medical community in the idea of TRT (even if that wasn't what Brown-Sequard called it).

What Do We Do for Low T Today?

Fast forward through more than 120 years of medical experimentation and advances since Charles-Edouard Brown-Sequard's self-injections, and you'll find yourself in a time (right now) where TRT offers many effective options for the treatment of Low Testosterone.

If you or your loved one has been diagnosed with Low T, you may be wondering if anything can be done, and if so, what? There's plenty of good news out there for men suffering from Low T. As this condition has received more attention over the past several decades, many medical advances have given Low T patients a variety of treatment options. When testosterone therapy began more than six decades ago, daily injections provided the only way to administer testosterone. Since that time, advances in this field have allowed healthcare providers to provide TRT in several ways.

In this chapter, I'd like to discuss the current methods of treatment for Low T; but first, let's take a look at some things you should know before you seek any kind of treatment, starting with the benefits of TRT.

Testosterone Replacement Therapy— What's In It for You?

Already we've learned about the symptoms of Low T, starting with its sexual varieties and moving through the mental/emotional and non-sexual physical ones. If Low T can cause so many physical and mental/emotional problems, then can we assume that replacing that lost testosterone through TRT might have as many *positive* effects?

Absolutely! Consider a few of the major benefits of testosterone replacement therapy:

- Improvement in sexual symptoms (libido, ability to maintain erections, etc.)
- Improvement in mental/emotional symptoms (energy, memory, concentration, mood, etc.)
- Improvement in physical symptoms
- Increased bone density
- Helps prevent Metabolic Syndrome (the combination of diabetes, high cholesterol, obesity, and high blood pressure)
- Correction of anemia
- May help to prevent Alzheimer's disease
- Cardioprotective (serving to protect the heart)
- Lowers cholesterol
- Lowers blood pressure
- Decreases fat and increases lean muscle mass

If testosterone replacement therapy has *that* many positive effects on a man with Low T, it might seem like a no-brainer that he'd sign up today. But before you and your loved one decide to take this path, consider several important issues.

Before You Decide … Talk to Your Doctor

Testosterone replacement therapy involves treatment with a steroid hormone, and any treatment with a steroid hormone presents certain risks—slight risks, in most cases—of certain side effects (more on those later). *That is why it is so important before you begin any form of testosterone replacement therapy to talk very candidly to your doctor about your own medical history and conditions.*

It is especially important to alert your doctor if you have or ever had prostate cancer or male breast cancer. For many years, doctors believed that testosterone replacement therapy increased a man's risk of prostate cancer. While no medical evidence proves that TRT causes prostate cancer, it is possible that if a patient has early prostate cancer, testosterone may stimulate the cancer's growth. For that reason, it is often recommended that men with prostate cancer should not take TRT in any form. Furthermore, all men considering TRT should undergo prostate screening before they begin therapy. Also, tell your doctor if you have any of the following medical conditions:

- Diabetes
- Sleep apnea
- Chronic breathing problems
- Liver disease
- Overweight

Once you have discussed your health history with your doctor, you can make a more informed choice on whether to pursue TRT, and if so, in what form.

Knowing the Risks … and the Side Effects

Because testosterone is a naturally occurring steroid hormone with a wide range of effects—some of them profound—it makes sense that the introduction of new testosterone into the bloodstream of an otherwise healthy man could present the risk of some side effects.

Testosterone replacement therapy does carry its share of risks and side effects. That is why it is so important to sit down with your doctor and get all the facts before you begin therapy.

Consider a few of the most common side effects:

1. **Increase in red blood cell count.** One of the most significant risks/side effects of testosterone replacement therapy, especially in older men, is an increase in red blood cells. This can be a good

thing for patients with anemia (low blood cell counts), but it can be very dangerous to others, because too much blood in the circulatory system can block blood vessels and cause potentially catastrophic events, such as strokes.

2. **Growth of the prostate gland.** Testosterone replacement therapy sometimes causes an increase in the size of the prostate gland. And if the patient already has an enlarged prostate, a condition called benign prostatic hyperplasia (BPH), testosterone may make the condition worse. That could lead to symptoms such as painful or difficult urination. This is especially true for men over 50 years of age. One other note: While no evidence shows that testosterone replacement therapy increases the risk of prostate cancer, men with a history of this disease should give special thought, along with their doctor, to the wisdom of testosterone therapy in their case.

3. **Skin reactions.** Men who use the testosterone patch may have some skin reactions. Those who use gels are less likely to have these symptoms. Skin reactions with the use of injections are very rare.

4. **Infertility.** A man's production of sperm depends on the natural production of testosterone in the testes. When "outside" testosterone gets introduced, the testes stop producing testosterone, which means sperm production slows way down or stops altogether. This can be a temporary or permanent side effect of TRT. This is an important consideration for men who still want to have a family. Some men have put off testosterone therapy until after they finish fathering children. Yet others who desire to preserve fertility are using Clomid, another option to safely raise T-levels.

5. **Sleep apnea.** Sleep apnea, a condition that causes sleepers to stop breathing for sometimes dangerously long periods of

time, is an uncommon side effect of testosterone therapy. Some reports indicate that increased testosterone levels may worsen already existing sleep apnea.

6. **Fluid retention.** This uncommon side effect of testosterone replacement therapy occurs mostly in older men. It can lead to leg or ankle swelling or an aggravation of high blood pressure or congestive heart failure.

7. **Enlargement or tenderness of the breasts.** This side effect can occur in older men and can be reversed by decreasing the testosterone dosage or adding an additional medicine to lower estrogen.

8. **Other possible side effects.** May include acne, oily skin, increased body hair, and flushing.

If you are considering testosterone replacement therapy, be aware that other risks/side effects may exist that, as yet, have not been documented. Talk with your doctor about any "new" side effects of testosterone replacement therapy.

Methods of Testosterone Therapy

While the prescribed treatment for Low T is most often testosterone replacement therapy, several delivery methods exist, each having their own advantages and disadvantages. Which one you choose depends on your preferences for the delivery method (for example, if you don't like needles, you may want to avoid the injection method), the side effects of each system, and, of course, the cost.

Once your doctor has diagnosed Low T, and once he or she has recommended TRT, it's time for you as a couple to discuss with your doctor which method is right for you. Let's consider the available methods of testosterone replacement therapy, starting with one that is strongly discouraged and almost never prescribed:

1. **Oral (Pills).** While neither I nor any other responsible health-care professional would recommend using testosterone replacement pills for most cases of Low T—in fact, we strongly discourage it—they do merit mention. Testosterone *is* available in pill form, but this method of treatment puts the patient at high risk of severe complications of the liver, specifically liver toxicity.

In some rare cases, physicians prescribe oral testosterone, but in these situations the symptoms and condition are severe enough to warrant the risk. For the overwhelming majority of men suffering from Low T, *testosterone pills are not prescribed or recommended.*

The one exception to this rule is a testosterone treatment called Andriol. But this drug has two significant problems: First, it's not generally available in the United States. Second, it's not as effective as the other treatment options.

The bottom line? Forget about treating Low T with pills—at least until someone develops one that is both safe and effective.

2. **Testosterone Injections**. This is one of the most cost-effective (about $30 per month) and convenient forms of testosterone replacement therapy in use today. It has also been around the longest—almost 70 years.

With this method, the patient receives an injection directly into a muscle, usually in the buttocks, about every two weeks. The patient can administer the shot himself or have a family member or friend do it. If no one at home feels comfortable giving an injection, then the patient can go to a doctor or nurse to receive it.

When doctors first began administering testosterone treatment, this was the only form of TRT available. In fact, in the 1940s, patients had to receive daily injections of a form of testosterone called *testosterone propionate*. Over the years, however, improvements in testosterone treatments have helped make injections a much more practical method of TRT. Longer-lasting testosterone treatments called *testosterone cypionate* and *testosterone enanthate* allow patients to receive injections far less frequently—about every one or two weeks, depending on the patient.

But testosterone injections have their own disadvantages, starting with the fact that the patient receives a "rush" of testosterone immediately after the injection, only to have his testosterone levels fall continuously until the next injection. As you might expect, this means swings in mood, energy level, and sex drive.

The other disadvantage is the need for the injections themselves. No matter what you might try to tell your children before they receive their annual flu shot, injections are painful. Not only that, it can be very inconvenient to make an appointment every one to two weeks to receive a testosterone injection.

3. **Buccal Cavity Treatment.** In this treatment, a product called "Striant," shaped like a pellet, is placed above the top teeth on the gum where it meets the upper lip (called the buccal cavity), where it adheres to the gum. It stays there all day, delivering testosterone through the gums. The testosterone doesn't seep into the saliva, and there is no danger of passing it on to another person during kissing. The pellet is replaced every 12 hours.

This method of treatment has been found to be very effective, but carries possible side effects such as pain, redness or irritation of the gums at the application site, a bitter taste in the mouth, changes in how food and drink taste, and headaches. The approximate cost of this form of treatment is $200-$500 per month.

4. **Transdermal Testosterone Delivery Systems (Patches).** Transdermal patches—patches that stick to the skin and deliver medicine into the bloodstream—have become popular methods for treatment of a variety of medical issues. Patches exist for trying to quit smoking (nicotine patches), birth control, the

treatment of menopause, pain relief, and more. And, of course, there are patches for the treatment of Low Testosterone.

Originally, the use of patches for TRT meant shaving the scrotum (try not to cringe too much; this has become unnecessary), attaching a testosterone patch to the freshly shaved skin, and then basically "gluing" it to that most sensitive part of the body with a hairdryer or other heat source.

If that were the only option, getting jabbed in the behind a few times a month doesn't sound so bad, does it?

Fortunately, advancements in "patch technology" have made such a painful process unnecessary. Now, the Low T patient can simply apply the patch (called Androderm) every day to his back, abdomen, upper arm, or thigh. From there, the patch releases the testosterone into his bloodstream through his skin.

Patches have a major advantage over injections in that they yield less of a "yo-yo" effect in the patient's testosterone level. The patch releases the medicine more uniformly, without giving the patient large spikes or drops in his testosterone level.

Disadvantages include the inability of some patients to absorb enough testosterone through their skin to elevate their testosterone to high enough levels. Another problem is skin reactions, which affect a fairly high percentage of men who use the patch. Finally, this is one of the more expensive methods of TRT on the market today. For those men whose skin can absorb enough testosterone to bring their levels up to adequate levels, however, the patch is an excellent way to go.

NOTE: Testosterone transdermal patches have been known to burn the skin at the application site during MRI (magnetic resonance imaging) examinations. To avoid that, simply remove the patch before undergoing an MRI.

5. **Transdermal Testosterone Gel (T-gel)**. Testosterone gels (T-gel) are the most common form of testosterone therapy used in the United States today. Testosterone gels account for about

60 percent of the testosterone replacement market. As of this writing, the United States Food and Drug Administration has approved four T-gels: Androgel, Testim, Fortesta, and Axiron (the new underarm gel).

These medications are very simple to use. Patients rub them into the skin daily, usually around the inner thighs or upper arms or shoulders. As the gel dries, the patient's body absorbs the testosterone through the skin and into the bloodstream, which helps his body reach normal testosterone levels.

Like the patch, this form of testosterone therapy is very expensive—approximately $200-$400 per month, although with an insurance copay it drops to $40-$60 per month—but it is very effective and is much less likely to cause skin reactions than patches. The gel is a very effective form of TRT, but does have some drawbacks. First, the user should not take a bath or shower for at least two hours after application. Second, some patients consider this a messy, inconvenient means of TRT.

Finally, consider some warnings for using these products: Women should *never* use testosterone gels. These medications can cause birth defects, so great care should be taken to make sure a pregnant woman never comes into contact with them. The medication also can be transmitted to your partner through skin-to-skin contact. To avoid this, avoid close contact until the gel completely dries, or cover the area where you applied the gel. If contact occurs, immediately wash with soap and water. Also take care to ensure that these gels do not come into contact with the skin of children.

6. **Testosterone Pellets.** In this method, your physician inserts testosterone pellets under the skin—usually above the buttocks—once every 3 to 6 months. The pellets release testosterone into the bloodstream slowly and steadily, very much like naturally occurring testosterone. For that reason, this method produces very few of the "peaks and valleys" associated

with injections and other forms of TRT. For the same reason, it carries fewer side effects than other treatment methods.

Only one testosterone replacement product—Testopel—exists in pellet form. This method of testosterone replacement appeals to many Low T patients because treatment is fairly simple: through a small incision in the skin and using a local anesthetic and a cannula (a tube used to insert the medication under the skin), a physician inserts the pellets (usually 6 or 8 at a time, about the size of a grain of rice). No patches, no creams, no injections! The patient has to remember only when the time comes for a new treatment (some studies have shown that pellets maintain the testosterone level for up to 4 months).

Some patients suffer minor discomfort or pain at the application site, especially the day after the implantation. And though it rarely happens, the pellets can resurface through the skin. The pellets also are very expensive—about $60 each—so this form of treatment carries a fairly high price tag.

A Final Note: Be Patient!

Suppose you and your loved one have talked to the doctor and have received a diagnosis of Low T. After more conversation, you've decided that testosterone replacement therapy is the best option for you. It's time, you say to one another, to do something about the sexual problems, the mood swings, the low energy, and his inability to think and concentrate.

In short, it's time to do something to get his mojo back!

Once you've decided which treatment is best for you, you probably will wonder, *How long after we start treatment will we start noticing improvements?*

Understand that the symptoms of Low T won't disappear, or even improve, overnight—or perhaps even within a few weeks or months. While a man's serum testosterone levels will improve relatively quickly, sometimes within one or two weeks after the beginning of therapy, the symptoms likely won't noticeably improve for two or three months, depending on the patient and the mode of treatment.

Most men suffering with Low T (as well as their loved ones) would love to take a "magic pill" that works as quickly and effectively as if they were taking a couple of Ibuprofen tablets for a headache. I'm sorry to have to say that many men don't see noticeable improvements in their symptoms for up to three months. Just as the symptoms came on gradually, so will the improvements. The positive effects on sex drive and mood will take about 90 days, while improvements in muscle mass and strength will appear in 90 to 180 days. Energy level is usually the first to improve, as quickly as one week in many patients.

If we're honest with ourselves, of course, we have to admit that we want results *right now*. All I can say is—sorry! Expect recovery from the symptoms of Low Testosterone to be a process rather than an event. As the two of you move through that process, do your best to remain patient with one another, supporting and encouraging each other.

Believe me, as one who has gone through the process, it's well worth the wait.

CHAPTER SIX

How Can We Find a Doctor?

For some time you've observed your partner's symptoms and listened to his complaints of low energy, lack of strength, and that persistent "down" feeling. You *know* something is wrong and you have come to suspect that it might be Low T (though, as pointed out earlier, many symptoms of Low T can point to any number of physical ailments). Perhaps you have even gently and lovingly suggested that it's time to see a doctor and to (gasp!) get your guy's testosterone level checked.

Once he agrees, then as soon as possible take the next step, so both of you can get some peace of mind. If the problem really is Low T, then you need to start considering treatment options.

While this part of the process of returning to wholeness might seem like the simplest of them all—you might be thinking, *How hard can it be to make an appointment to get checked for Low T? We'll just call the family doctor and get this process started!*— it's not always as simple as making an appointment and showing up for it. So let's briefly walk through the process.

Pick Your Family Practioner's Brain

For most of us, the place to begin is obvious: With our family practitioner. Probably you've known him or her for many years. You feel comfortable with each other. This "general practioner" knows you well, which can be an important consideration when discussing the more personal symptoms of Low T.

But how can you know if your family physician knows enough about Low T to provide you with the help you need?

Come prepared to your appointment to ask some very pointed questions about Low T and what your doctor may know about it. Probably you'll want to make an appointment for a "sit down" discussion, so you can pick your doc's brain a bit. Since Low Testosterone can lead to a long list of serious conditions, don't feel even a little hesitant about discovering how "up-to-date" your doctor is about Low T.

What sort of questions should you ask? I recommend that you come with a list that can help you kill two birds with one stone, so to speak. Your questions should uncover not only how much your doctor knows about Low T, but also should give you the opportunity to acquire the information you'll need to make informed decisions on treatment options. Make sure you ask the kinds of questions that will answer the following basic questions:

- *What does the doctor know about Low T, and what kind of symptoms should he or she be looking for?* It's fortunate these days that Low T is getting a higher profile, even on television, where several commercials have popped up to talk about the condition. If you're having a hard time getting the ball rolling, perhaps you could mention that you've seen one of these ads and then observe how the doctor responds.

- *Does the doctor have a good idea of the necessary blood tests?* Testing for Low T requires specialized blood tests, and not all doctors are up-to-date on which tests to use. It is important for the doctor to check both a Free and Total Testosterone; your physician also needs to know how to interpret the results.

- *Does the doctor know about the various treatment options for Low T and how to administer them?* Even now, at the beginning of the second decade of the new millennium, many doctors either know little about Low T or subscribe to outdated and disproven ideas about it. Some of the medical science about Low T is so new that many in the medical community haven't yet caught up with it.

- *Is the doctor willing to prescribe testosterone treatment if the problem really turns out to be Low T?* Testosterone treatment is very safe, especially when a doctor oversees the treatment (a given). What possible side effects exist, tend to be minimal. A surprising number of doctors, however—especially family or general practitioners—feel reluctant or unwilling to prescribe testosterone replacement therapy (TRT), even for textbook cases of Low T. Many doctors simply aren't up-to-date on medical knowledge of Low T and how to treat it. In order to avoid any misunderstandings, therefore, ask this question up front, and don't be afraid to ask it directly.

At the same time, consider several other questions to ask your doctor. "Do you treat many patients with Low T? And if not, can you refer me to someone who does?" "How do you diagnose Low T?" "Do you check both for Free and Total Testosterone?"

Finding a Specialist

After your appointment, you may discover that your family doctor cannot offer you the help you need. If your questions don't yield the necessary answers, then you may want to request a referral to a urologist, a doctor who specializes in the urinary tract and in the male reproductive system. Please don't worry about hurting your family doctor's feelings—true professionals don't get offended when you ask for a referral.

While a general practitioner or family doctor may or may not possess the most up-to-date information on Low T, a urologist should be able to answer all of your questions, make an accurate diagnosis, and prescribe the treatment you or your partner needs. At the very least, every urologist should be more knowledgeable and a lot more up-to-date on the latest trends and findings associated with the treatment of Low T than most general practitioners can be.

If for some reason your family doctor can't recommend a urologist, then you may have to do a little detective work to find one in your area. The Yellow Pages can be a good tool, and for those with Internet connections, the Web offers several resources for locating a local urologist's office. You might check out one of several excellent online resources for finding a urologist, such as UrologyHealth.org, which uses a zip code search for urologists who are sanctioned members of the American Urological Association (AUA), the top professional association for urologists.

Once you find a suitable specialist and make an appointment, be aware that your first visit might be more of a "getting to know you" meeting than a diagnostic session. Remember, treating Low T is a process and not an event; you'll probably be spending a lot of time at your urologist's office, especially in the beginning, as he tracks your progress and the possible side effects of testosterone replacement therapy.

Also, most men get very uncomfortable talking about the symptoms of Low T, at least at first. If you can find a urologist who has just the right "bedside manner" for you, you'll be that much further ahead in getting your problem diagnosed and treated. For these reasons, make sure you feel comfortable with your choice of urologist.

This first meeting can also be a good time to find out about the urologist's credentials—his training, his familiarity and experience with Low T symptoms, and his experiences treating other men with the same problem. As you move past that first appointment, you (and your partner) should have ample opportunity to ask your urologist questions about Low T and how he likes to treat it.

Consider several questions you might want to ask on your first visit to the urologist's office:

- How can we know for sure that it's Low T?
- Which treatment is best for us and why?
- What are the benefits of TRT?
- How long will it likely take before we see the benefits of TRT?
- How can we lessen or avoid the side effects of TRT?
- Should we do anything else to help the testosterone do its work?
- What happens if the first treatment doesn't work?

Wondering What to Tell Your Urologist? Try *Everything!*

Let's close this chapter with what I consider to be very sound advice. Men, don't feel afraid, ashamed, or embarrassed to tell your urologist *everything*. That includes the sexual dysfunction you may be experiencing.

Now, I know that no man likes talking about that sort of thing. I didn't, and I don't know why you would, either. The truth is, most of us associate our sex drive and ability to perform sexually with manhood itself—at least, a very big part of it. So we feel uncomfortable discussing it. But *leaving out* that crucial bit of information can seriously hamper successful treatment of your condition.

Don't forget that a urologist is a trained, experienced medical professional who probably has diagnosed and treated scores of men with symptoms just like yours—or even worse. *Nothing* you tell him will surprise or shock him….and I truly mean Nothing. Nor is he going to judge you or look down on you as "less of a man" because you suffer from the symptoms of Low T. The point is to get you well and functioning as you want to; and to do that, he needs to know *everything* that might have relevance to your condition.

Think of it this way. If your car started to sputter and and lurch and belch black smoke every time you came to a stop sign or red light, would you feel afraid to tell your mechanic about it, for fear that he might consider you less of a man for not knowing how to fix it? I doubt it. He has knowledge that you probably lack, and he's probably encountered this problem before. So you wouldn't likely tell him, "Um, well, my car has been having a little trouble lately. But I really don't want to tell you what sort of trouble. I hope you understand." If you want the car fixed, you'll tell him everything you've noticed.

In a similar way, a urologist needs to know all of your symptoms. As a specialist in this field, he understands better than anyone, including other medical professionals, one of the main points I want to make in this book: *A man who suffers from Low T isn't any less of a man than he's ever been; he just has a medical condition that needs to be treated.* Fortunately, it's a condition that lends itself very well to treatment. And the results can be dramatic.

If you don't talk to your urologist about your symptoms—*all* of your symptoms—then you'll just make it that much more difficult to get a diagnosis and treatment for your Low T. In fact, if you hold back on describing your symptoms, it's possible you may not get a correct diagnosis at all. So why risk it? No matter what lie that little voice in your head may tell you about some mythical "loss of manhood," tell your urologist everything. If you have to plow through embarrassment, then plow through it. Just get the help you need.

Who knows? You might find that your urologist is just like me: A licensed, highly trained doctor who is also a patient undergoing treatment—quite successfully!—for the common medical condition known as Low T.

Did I tell you that I recently finished an Ironman triathlon?

Not that I'm competitive, or anything.

CHAPTER SEVEN

What Should We Expect?

How Treatment for Low T Might Play Out

Mary had noticed the changes in her husband, Sam, and they concerned her. In fact, the word *concerned* probably didn't do her thoughts and feelings justice. Her husband wasn't himself lately, and she was becoming very frustrated and increasingly worried … even alarmed.

From what she could see, even those small "bumps in the road" that life always seems to bring had ruffled him in ways that never had before. The normally even-tempered gentleman she had spent most of her life with had become a bit of a hothead, and at the slightest irritations. Though Sam always had been a "people person," he had become increasingly short-tempered with everyone, including those he loved most. Even their beloved grandchildren, the little boy and girl he had doted over, had become the objects of his outbursts. Sam also had become very moody—at times overly passive, and at other times unusually aggressive. Finally, Sam complained frequently about his fatigue and lack of physical stamina.

Mary found all of these changes difficult to take; she never knew what kind of mood would rule Sam from day to day. Sometimes she found it very difficult to approach him at all.

And their sex life? Over time, it had become more like *what sex life?* Mary and Sam once had enjoyed a healthy, even passionate sex life. But now the lack of sexual intimacy in their marriage made her wonder (as with so many women in this situation) what was wrong with *her*. She missed the closeness that sexual intimacy provides. The way she saw it, they weren't living like husband and wife anymore, but more like two acquaintances sleeping in the same room.

Sam just wasn't himself—and in more ways than Mary liked thinking about. A horrible thought haunted her as she pondered the changes she'd seen in Sam. *Are these the early signs of Alzheimer's disease?* She knew a little about that awful condition, as a few of her family members had suffered and died from Alzheimer's. As much as Sam had changed over the past few years, however, she still loved him deeply, and she couldn't bear the thought of seeing her husband deteriorate mentally and physically as Alzheimer's disease ravaged his mind and body.

One day, the subject of a daytime talk show caught Mary's attention: Low Testosterone, a medical condition she knew nothing about. The show included the "expert," a urologist who specialized in the treatment of Low T, as well as a couple of Low T patients and their wives. As she listened to what one of the women said about her own husband's symptoms, it almost felt as though she were listening to herself.

That sounds just like Sam! she thought.

Mary listened attentively and then mentally went through a checklist of the symptoms she'd heard described on the show:

Temperamental and moody? Yeah, that was Sam! She thought about how in previous years she never could have imagined this gentle, mild-mannered man reacting the way he had to such small problems. Life at home had started to feel like a bit of a roller coaster ride.

Lacking any desire for sexual intimacy? Mary almost couldn't remember the last time she and Sam had shared a night of intimacy. It seemed that Sam, a man who'd had a very healthy appetite for sex, just had no interest anymore.

Lacking physical strength and stamina? His words, not hers! She had noticed that Sam oftentimes didn't want to do anything but stay at home, sleeping or watching TV. And this from a man who had been an outstanding athlete in his younger years and who always had enjoyed being active!

Mary felt some small sense of encouragement when she heard the doctor on the talk show say that Low T was a very treatable medical condition and that many men who receive treatment live normal, healthy lives.

Before she had watched the talk show, Mary knew next to nothing about testosterone. Like most people, she knew men had the substance floating around in their bodies and that it had something to do with why most men seemed to want sex most of the time. Other than that, she barely knew how to say "testosterone," let alone what it did.

The more Mary thought about Sam's symptoms, the more she became sure that this otherwise healthy man suffered from a lack of testosterone. She didn't understand how the stuff worked or how it got into a man's bloodstream; she just knew everything she'd seen in her husband pointed to Low T.

And now the question: What would she do about it?

What Next?

Mary missed the man Sam used to be, and she felt determined to try just about anything to encourage him to see a doctor to learn if Low T really was the problem. *If I can just get him to see a doctor and get some help, then maybe he can become the same Sam I've known for all these years!* she thought. *But how do I approach him to talk about what I just heard on the talk show?*

Finally, Mary decided to approach Sam gently but directly to talk to him about low testosterone. At first, Sam—like so many men when they hear the suggestion that they may have Low T—resisted. But as Mary, with tears in her eyes, persisted, Sam agreed to let her make an appointment with a urologist to have his testosterone levels checked.

Sam didn't want to admit it—to Mary or to anyone else—but his initial reluctance to see a doctor had more to do with his general discomfort with doctors than anything else. He hadn't often visited the family doctor, and when he had, it usually represented a last-resort attempt to get over a bad case of the flu or bronchitis.

But now Sam felt doubly uncomfortable with seeing the doctor. He didn't know exactly what a urologist did, but just the word *urologist* made him think of being touched and handled "down there." And the thought of having to talk about the sex part of the whole thing—*that* made Sam's stomach hurt. He had a hard enough time talking about sexual issues with his wife, and he'd made love with her more times than either of them could count. And now, he'd be talking about his loss of sex drive to a man who was, at least to this point, a *complete stranger*.

In the days leading up to his appointment, Sam became more and more anxious about what was about to happen—what the doctor would do and what he would have to talk about. For days, he didn't say much to Mary about his thoughts, fears, and anxiety. But finally, as they lay in bed on the eve of his appointment, he opened up to his wife.

"Honey, you watched that TV show about Low T," he reminded her. "What kinds of tests do you think the doctor will do on me tomorrow?"

"I'm not sure about that," she answered, still not aware that Sam felt uncomfortable talking about the subject and that he felt very worried about what awaited him the next day. Then it dawned on Mary; her husband felt *really* worried about his appointment. She had become so preoccupied with getting him well—and of getting back the Sam she'd known and loved all those years—that she hadn't given much thought to how Sam felt about the whole thing.

Mary felt a small twinge of guilt for not thinking about that part of their story. So instead of simply telling him not to worry and then going to sleep, Mary offered some tender, loving words of encouragement: "Sam, I don't want you to worry. I'll be right there with you tomorrow, and we'll get through this together. It's going to be fine, you'll see!"

That did make Sam feel better. He wasn't sure why, but it did. His worries and fears began to fade, and his stomach stopped churning. He leaned over and kissed his wife goodnight, then rolled over onto his side with his pillow under his head. He slept better that night than he had all week.

The Appointment: What to Expect

Many men looking at their first visit to a urologist—especially when they know they're going to be checked for Low T—feel a sense of anxiety. That's only natural whenever we face a lot of unknowns.

What follows are some things you can expect as you begin this journey toward wholeness and wellness. While every patient, every partner, and every doctor is different, the following provides a general look at the steps you'll take once you've made that important decision to take your mate and his symptoms to a medical professional who specializes in treating Low T.

First, the nurse will check you in and take your vitals—blood pressure, heart rate, weight, temperature—and will give you a questionnaire to answer.

When I see a patient for the first time, I always introduce myself and then ask, "what brings you in to see me," or "how can I help you?"

The doctor will listen to your responses, take a medical history (the nurse generally takes down most of this information when you first arrive) and do a physical exam of your entire body—including the dreaded rectal exam, to check the health of the prostate.

At the end of the first appointment, a nurse or technician will draw some blood; results normally take a week to come back. I usually arrange a follow up visit for one to two weeks later to discuss the results. At that time I also explain thoroughly the risks and benefits of TRT, draw more blood if needed, and start testosterone injections or give a prescription for another method of TRT. If the patient chooses injections, I see him one week after the first shot; if he chooses the gel, I see him three weeks later.

The Blood Test

Since many of the symptoms of Low T are similar or identical to several other physical problems, the only way to know for sure is through a simple blood test.

Blood tests check for several things. One tests for both free and total testosterone, to screen for Low T; another kind of test (PSA) screens for prostate cancer; a third kind (TSH) checks for proper thyroid function; and a final one (hemoglobin and hematocrit) looks for anemia and gets a baseline blood count.

Any abnormal test results can confirm Low T or some other problem that can cause similar symptoms. In general, the diagnosis of Low T takes less than one week after receiving back the results from the blood test. Clinically speaking, any patient with symptoms of Low T who has a Total T less than 400 ng/dl *or* a Free T less than 12 pg/ml is diagnosed with Low T.

Choosing a Treatment

In my practice, I encourage patients diagnosed with Low T to use a topical gel if they have good drug coverage on their insurance plan. If a three-week trial of the gel fails to start benefitting them, or fails to increase their serum T levels, then I recommend injection therapy. If the patient is going to pay out of pocket for his medications, then I usually recommend the injections, because they are the cheapest method. Alternatively, I recommend having a local compounding pharmacy make a topical cream to apply to the skin daily.

The Prognosis

Almost 100 percent of men get their T levels therapeutic or back to normal within three months of seeing me after their initial visit; most men do so much sooner than that. Once their blood levels return to normal, within three months they begin to see the maximum benefit from the treatment, which should last a lifetime, so long as they continue using the medication.

Normal. Maximum benefit. For a lifetime. Doesn't that sound worth a few moments of possible uneasiness at the doctor's office?

CHAPTER EIGHT

Who's at Risk?

The Risk Factors of Low T and What to Do About Them

At least one "risk factor" for Low T all of us want to avoid, but none of us can—at least, not so long as we manage to stay alive. Can you guess it? It's aging (see chapter 11). So at the risk of stating the *incredibly* obvious, let me point out that aging is something we all do, if we're fortunate enough to keep breathing. As we age, our testosterone levels *will* fall.

So the short answer to the question of whose testosterone levels will drop, is

"Any man who ages."

A fall in our testosterone levels as we age—along with the related decline in sex drive (most men over forty certainly don't have the libidos they had in their twenties) and the changes in our bodies (some loss of muscle mass and definition)—is perfectly normal and natural, even desirable in some ways. But a man who lacks a normal amount of testosterone in his bloodstream *for his age* suffers from a testosterone deficiency.

Many factors besides aging can put a man at risk for testosterone deficiency. Some of them are medical (injuries and illnesses), some are genetic/developmental (the "inherited" disorders or syndromes), and others have to do with lifestyle choices. While a man can't control all the factors that make him a candidate for Low T (we'll look at the factors he can control), simply knowing about the risk factors can provide a giant step forward in diagnosing and treating this condition.

Injuries, Illnesses, and Some Medical Treatments

The human body is an amazing collection of systems that work together to keep a man healthy and functioning at an optimal level. When one or more of those systems malfunctions, due to injury or illness, lowered testosterone levels can result. Consider some of the problems that can occur through injury or illness.

Damage to the testicles or scrotum. The testicles, the primary producers of testosterone in the male body, hang outside the body cavity within the scrotum. They do so in order to stay at a slightly lower temperature than the rest of the body, which enables them to produce sperm.

The downside of this design is that the testicles are vulnerable to injury, which can lead to Low Testosterone. When the testicles get damaged, they may not produce the amount of testosterone a man needs for optimal health. Injury to the testicles does not automatically mean a lower testosterone level; sometimes injured testicles, or even one healthy testicle, still produce satisfactory amounts of testosterone.

Cirrhosis of the liver. This condition is one of the most important of all medical risk factors for Low Testosterone, because the liver destroys female sex hormones. When the liver stops functioning properly, a buildup of female sex hormones can develop in the man's bloodstream, leading to (among other things) testicular atrophy, or a shrinkage of the testicles.

This progressive disease develops over a long period of time. It replaces healthy liver cells with scar tissue, which blocks the flow of blood through the liver. The best-known cause of cirrhosis of the liver is alcohol abuse, but many things can cause it, including an infection of Hepatitis C, a buildup of toxic metals in the bloodstream, some viruses, and autoimmune liver disease, a condition in which the body's immune system attacks the liver.

Kidney failure. The kidneys make up part of the body's excretory system; they filter out impurities in the blood. When the kidneys fail, serious health complications result. One of those complications causes the pituitary gland to overproduce the hormone prolactin, best known for aiding in lactation—the production of breast milk. In the male body, too-high levels of prolactin interfere with the production of testosterone.

Cancer and cancer treatments. Testicular cancers and other cancer treatments can lead to lowered testosterone production. Chemotherapy and radiation therapy, commonly used to treat many forms of cancer, can have the same effect, because both can damage the Leydig cells in the testicles, which produce testosterone. Sometimes, the cells damaged through chemotherapy and radiation therapy recover, allowing testosterone production to return to normal. Sometimes, however, the damage is irreversible, meaning the patient's body will not produce enough testosterone.

Treatment for prostate cancer also leads to lower testosterone; in fact, one of the treatments for this disease is to take steps to *lower* testosterone levels. That is because most prostate cancer cannot grow without a small amount of testosterone.

Hypertension (high blood pressure). High blood pressure, which affects close to 100 million Americans, has been called the "silent killer" because it produces few if any noticeable symptoms and because it can cause heart attacks, heart disease, strokes, kidney failure, and other life-threatening medical conditions.

The relationship between high blood pressure and erectile dysfunction is well known. But some recent studies have shown that men with hypertension seem to have lower levels of testosterone than those who don't.

Infectious diseases. We usually think of mumps as a childhood disease, and most of the time that's true. If a human male contracts this infection during adolescence or early adulthood, however, the long-term damage may include Low Testosterone production. That happens when the infection causes inflammation of the testes.

The HIV/AIDS virus also can lower levels of testosterone because it affects the hypothalamus, pituitary, and testes. Other diseases, such as meningitis and syphilis, can also lead to lower testosterone levels.

Diabetes. In recent years, it has become more and more clear that a very real relationship exists between diabetes and Low T. While it's not clear if one condition causes the other, studies in the past decade have shown that men with type 2 diabetes are much more likely to suffer from Low Testosterone. In 2007, a study of 100 men with type-2 diabetes at the State University of New York at Buffalo found that one-third of the study's participants also had Low Testosterone.

Injury or disease of the pituitary gland or hypothalamus. Damage to the pituitary gland and/or hypothalamus can cause Low T because the pituitary, hypothalamus, and testicles all work together to produce testosterone and get it flowing into the bloodstream. A healthy hypothalamus produces gonadotropin releasing hormone (GnRH), which triggers the healthy pituitary gland's production of luteinizing hormone (LH). The LH then travels to the testicles, signaling them to produce testosterone. Tumors of the pituitary also can lead to the overproduction of prolactin, which suppresses sex hormone levels.

Genetic and Developmental Risk Factors

Some things in life remain out of our control, and genetic and developmental disorders belong on that list. But as the old saying goes, to be forewarned is to be forearmed, and if you know or suspect that your loved one may suffer from one of the disorders listed below, you will move a step closer to fighting the battle against Low T.

Hemochromatosis. This relatively common genetic disorder affects an estimated two million Americans and causes the body to absorb too much dietary iron. The excess iron can settle in bodily organs, including the hypothalamus, pituitary gland, and the testicles, causing reduced testosterone production.

Klinefelter's syndrome. This genetic condition causes a deficiency in the production of testosterone. The medical community believes it affects between 1 in 500 and 1 in 1,000 men. About one in 500 men have the extra X chromosome, but show no symptoms of Klinefelter's syndrome.

The symptoms of Klinefelter's usually don't show up until puberty, when most boys experience the rush of testosterone that helps them develop into young men. These boys' bodies don't produce the increased amount of testosterone that the bodies of most of their peers do, and so they usually develop sparse or no body or facial hair, have little muscle definition, and may have enlarged breasts. Most fully-grown men with this syndrome have smaller-then-normal testicles, and many are infertile and cannot father children without medical help.

Kallmann syndrome. In this condition, the hypothalamus doesn't develop normally, which leads to a risk for Low Testosterone. In men with Kallmann syndrome, the underdeveloped hypothalamus doesn't release enough GnRH, leading to the underproduction of testosterone.

Cryptorchidism (undescended testicles). The testicles of the average man began developing inside his abdomen while an infant in his mother's womb. Shortly before birth, they drop into the scrotum. But in about 1 in 20 boys who are born at full term (about 260 days), and about 1 in 4 who are born premature, the testicles don't descend when they should. This condition usually corrects itself within the first year of life, but when it doesn't, the testicles may not develop fully. That can lead to deficiencies in testosterone production.

Prader-Willi syndrome. This rare genetic disorder is characterized by, among other things, Low Testosterone levels. Other symptoms of PWS are an extreme, insatiable appetite for food—which sometimes leads to extreme obesity—and undescended testicles.

Lifestyle-Related Risk Factors

While many risk factors of Low T lie beyond our control, several are related to lifestyle choices, which most certainly we can control. Consider some of the most significant:

Overweight/Obesity. We've already seen that one of the symptoms of Low Testosterone is unexplained weight gain. Well, it works the other way around, too. Excessive weight has been linked to the development of Low T in some men.

Here's how that works: Some of a man's testosterone is converted inside the body to estrogen, the female sex hormone. Just as women need smaller amounts of testosterone in their bodies than men do, so men need lower levels of estrogen than do women. Excess weight becomes a problem because that conversion from testosterone to estrogen takes place in the fat cells. So the more fat a man carries on his body, the more testosterone his body converts into estrogen. That, of course, leads to lower testosterone levels.

Obesity is epidemic in America, due mostly to the combination of poor diet and sedentary lifestyles. Today, nearly two-thirds of American adults are considered overweight, with about half of them considered obese. This problem doesn't result merely in a lot of "fat and happy" people; it results in countless preventable medical conditions, some of them very serious, even fatal. That includes hypertension, diabetes, as well as heart disease and some forms of cancer.

The possibility of developing Low T is yet another reason to do all you can to keep off those excess pounds.

Poor diet. If one risk for testosterone deficiency appears common to a majority of Americans, it's a poor diet. We are blessed with plenty to eat, but frankly, a lot of what we *do* eat was never meant for human consumption. We pack our grocery store shelves with all kinds of processed foods, preservatives and other additives, and items created using unnatural—and potentially destructive—methods.

What's more, the easy availability of "fast food" makes it far more convenient for us to hit the drive through and order the McWendy's Three-Quarter Pound Triple Cheeseburger—with the Salty Fries, of course—than to go to the time and effort it takes to fix a healthy meal.

Consuming a lot of junk food—foods high in sugar, transfats, corn syrup, and bleached white flour—not only causes weight gain, but also causes a man's testosterone levels to take a major dip.

Zinc deficiency. Poor diet often leads to zinc deficiency, but this condition merits special mention for two reasons: First, it has become very common in the United States, and second, zinc is extremely important for sexual function and for the production of testosterone. Some studies have shown that if a man suffers from Low T, there's a very good chance he also suffers from zinc deficiency.

What does zinc have to do with testosterone levels in men? A healthy level of dietary zinc lowers the body's levels of an enzyme called aromatase, which helps to convert testosterone into estrogen. On the other hand, a too-low level of dietary zinc over-activates this enzyme, which can throw the man's testosterone/estrogen balance out of whack. Also, an adequate level of dietary zinc helps in the production of the hormones responsible for telling the body to increase testosterone production.

Certain drugs/medications. At any given time, close to two-thirds of Americans use some kind of drug or medication; many of those drugs can affect our sex drive and testosterone levels. Some of the worst offenders are antidepressants like Prozac, Valium, and Elavil, and antihistamines like Benadryl, Antivert, and Dramamine. Painkillers such as Demerol, Codeine, and Oxycontin also present risks of lowered testosterone. Even commonly used over-the-counter medications such as Tagamet, Zantac, Pepcid AC, and Ibuprofen are believed to lower testosterone levels in men.

Smoking. How many good reasons exist to stop smoking—or never to start? Tobacco use is the leading cause of preventable death (through lung and other cancers, as well as cardiovascular disease) in the United States.

Add the higher risk of Low T to the list. Disagreement exists within the medical community about the relationship between cigarette smoking and Low T, but since smoking is unquestionably linked to high blood pressure—a known risk factor for Low T—a link does exist between the two, if an indirect one. Many experts also believe that the poison ingested by cigarette smokers can have a direct and negative affect on the Leydig cells in the testicles, which, again, help to create testosterone.

Stress. Although everyone goes through times of stress, I would argue that much of our stress comes not so much from life situations as to how we *react* to those situations.

The body responds to stress, in part, by releasing an increased amount of the hormone cortisol, also known as the "stress hormone." Cortisol is important to our health for many reasons, including the release of insulin, blood pressure regulation, and the body's ability to heal itself. Cortisol also helps to regulate our "fight or flight" instinct.

We need cortisol; without it, we couldn't survive. But an overproduction of cortisol, due to excess stress, can decrease the body's ability to produce testosterone. Why? In order to produce more cortisol, our bodies have to shut down or decrease other functions, if only temporarily. One of those affected functions is the production of testosterone. The more we can learn to relax and let things roll off our backs, the more efficiently our bodies produce the testosterone we need.

Lack of exercise/too much exercise. Proper exercise has an amazing number of positive effects on the body. It can strengthen and maintain the cardiovascular system, help in burning fat, and keep the muscles strong and toned. It also causes your body to release human growth hormone and testosterone into your blood stream. Contrary to this, a sedentary lifestyle can increase the risk of suffering from Low T, especially when it leads to excess weight gain.

On the other hand, excessive amounts of exercise can have a negative effect on testosterone levels. Why this should be so has prompted a lot of recent study and debate, but it has been shown that endurance trainers, marathoners, and distance cyclists sometimes have lower testosterone levels than less-active or non-active men their same age category.

Lack of sleep. At some point, we've all had to "burn the candle at both ends." When we don't get enough sleep, we feel tired, burned out, irritable, and physically weak. If we continue to deprive ourselves of sleep, we can become physically sick. But did you know that a chronic lack of sleep can have a devastating effect on a man's testosterone levels? Several dependable studies have shown a direct relationship between sack time and testosterone levels—the less sleep a man gets, the lower his testosterone level is likely to be.

A typical man's testosterone levels change during the course of a day, peaking early in the morning and then steadily decreasing to their lowest point in the evening. Getting enough sleep each night—seven or eight hours is about right for most men—is one way a man can help his body naturally raise its testosterone level. It's a fairly complicated process that has been compared to an IV drip of testosterone taking place during sleep. The more uninterrupted sleep a man gets, the more testosterone his body will produce.

Excessive alcohol use. Many studies have shown that drinking in moderation—a glass or two of wine with dinner, or a few beers with his friends—can have positive physical effects. But overdoing it can devastate our bodies. One of those ill effects is Low T.

Studies of men who drink heavily have shown that alcohol inhibits the production of testosterone and other male reproductive/sex hormones. Alcohol can play havoc on your endocrine system (the glands that produce the hormones your body needs to function properly), which causes your testicles to stop producing testosterone. One night of drinking to excess can reduce testosterone production for twenty-four hours; the effect worsens the more the man "binges."

Alcohol, when used to excess, increases and speeds up the removal of testosterone from the bloodstream and also decreases the production of testosterone by increasing the release of cortisol, the stress hormone. It also has a negative impact on the Leydig cells. Also, excessive alcohol use can cause weight gain, another risk factor for Low T. And severe cases of alcohol abuse can lead to cirrhosis of the liver, which also can lead to Low T.

Marijuana use. Debate rages today in the United States and elsewhere over the merits of legalizing marijuana. While I have no interest in getting into that argument here, I do want to point out that several studies have shown that the use of marijuana can lead to reduced libido, erectile dysfunction, decreased sperm production, and Low Testosterone. One study showed that smoking just one joint can suppress the body's output of testosterone, if only for a short while.

Performance-enhancing drug (anabolic steroids) use. A few decades ago, a public service blitz warned against the use of performance-enhancing drugs, substances which bodybuilders and athletes often took to make them stronger or faster. Anabolic steroids are basically synthetic versions of testosterone.

It is now a medically settled fact that the use of these drugs comes with some frightening side effects, including shrunken testicles and reduced testosterone production. The reason is fairly simple: When a man introduces anabolic steroids into his body, his endocrine system is "fooled" into cutting down on the natural production of testosterone.

Short-term use of these drugs usually means short-term reduction in natural testosterone production; long-term use can result in irrevocable damage.

Being married or in a committed relationship. You didn't read that incorrectly! We've all heard how married men, or those in a monogamous, long-term relationship, tend to be healthier and happier then those who "go solo." You might think part of that health and happiness would be a higher testosterone level.

You'd be wrong.

Recent research has shown conclusively that men in committed relationships (it doesn't seem to matter whether it's marriage or a long-term, monogamous relationship) tend to have significantly lower testosterone levels than unattached men of the same age groups. Researchers aren't entirely sure why married or "attached" men have lower testosterone, but one theory suggests that the man's body reacts to his relational state by producing less testosterone because he is no longer in a state of "hunting" for a mate. The lower levels of testosterone among married men also may keep them from straying, according to some research.

Even though being married or in a committed relationship can cause a drop in a man's testosterone level, the physical and emotional benefits of marriage—which have been proven and demonstrated—far outweigh the risk of slightly lower testosterone.

Attention new Dads! A recent study conducted on 624 men at Northwestern University concluded that becoming a new father can drop your testosterone levels by as much as 34%. It is not clear if the testosterone levels eventually come back to normal.

Keep the Testosterone Flowing

So what should you do to keep from becoming a front-running candidate for Low T—or to help your body begin producing testosterone if the levels aren't where they should be? I see two ways of approaching the information I've presented so far: preventive (keeping normal testosterone levels from dropping) and reparative (bringing testosterone levels up for someone who already has Low T).

You can't do anything to reduce some risk factors for Low T. You can't do anything to avoid the genetic or developmental issues that cause testosterone deficiency, and you can't undo accidents and injuries that may have led to reduced testosterone levels.

Many of these risk factors, however, are at least partially under your control. You *can* do something about your weight, about your physical condition, about the amount of quality sleep you get, and what you eat. And, of course, you can cut out the smoking (of cigarettes and marijuana alike) and the excessive drinking.

Everything I just listed is part of a healthy lifestyle, testosterone or no testosterone. Knowing that—and knowing at least something about the interconnectedness of so many of our bodily systems—it only makes sense that a healthy lifestyle can help keep your testosterone level where it needs to be. And making some changes may even help sufferers of Low T to regain their testosterone production.

Consider several things you can do to help prevent a drop in your testosterone levels, and perhaps help in recovery for those with Low T.

Drop Some Weight—But Don't Be in a Rush

If you (or your partner) is like a lot of men, you've probably thought about how to drop some of that unsightly ring of fat hanging from your midsection (and maybe other places). Many men tend to procrastinate, and one of the areas where we apply the "never do today what you can put off until tomorrow" strategy is weight loss.

People at a "right weight" for their height and build look and feel better, can take part in activities that overweight people cannot, and reduce the odds that they will develop potentially life-threatening conditions. So if your physical appearance and better general health don't provide you with enough motivation, then perhaps a potential boost in your testosterone level might push you toward the effort it takes to lose weight.

As you prepare to lose weight, understand that it's always better to take a slow-and-steady approach. Before you and your partner decide to put you on a crash diet and lose fifty pounds in two months, slow down! Being in too much of a hurry to trim down is counterproductive to anyone's general health, because cutting calorie intake too drastically causes the brain to go into "starvation mode." That is, your brain will begin to tell your body that it's starving. Your mind knows you have plenty of food available, but your body sees a famine going on, and therefore you need to keep some reserves. So to compensate for a sudden, self-imposed loss of nourishment, the brain sends a message to your testicles (and other glands) telling them to slow down or stop testosterone production—at least until the famine has passed. And when the testosterone isn't flowing like it should, your body doesn't burn body fat as efficiently as it would if you simply cut back moderately on your caloric intake and got some exercise.

So *do* lose weight—but don't give in to the temptation to use "fad diets" or starvation techniques to do it. Ask your doctor for some help in this area. He or she can point you in the right direction toward a local nutrition class or other resources. Susan and I revamped our nutrition strategy about the same time that I discovered I had Low T. Our diet consists mostly of low carbohydrate foods with an emphasis on proteins and vegetables. We basically avoid anything that our body turns into sugar, such as breads, rice, potatoes, and pasta. This has helped us to maintain our weight over the last 10 years.

Get off the Couch and Get Your Body Moving

Exercise isn't exactly a panacea, but it's pretty close. Regular exercise has an amazing array of positive effects on our bodies and minds. When we get enough of the right kind of exercise, we feel better, look better, and think more clearly, even as we tone up and lose some of that flab.

While it seems to make sense that regular exercise can increase a man's testosterone levels, the jury is still out on that one—at least, in the long term. Some studies seem to show that regular exercise can raise testosterone levels, while others are inconclusive or show no or little effect. But since we know about the healthy effects of regular exercise, it certainly can't hurt to make this part of your daily life.

One important note: It's always a good idea to visit your doctor before you start any exercise routine. Get a physical first, just to make sure your body is healthy enough to begin these activities or to increase the amount of exercise you get during the course of a week. I also suggest visiting a local fitness club and using a personal trainer to help get you on a plan tailored to your individual needs.

Three types of exercise should become a part of your efforts to get in shape: Flexibility exercises, cardiovascular exercise, and resistance exercise.

1. *Flexibility exercise.* Unfortunately, this is a too-often neglected part of many exercise routines. We have a lot to do each day, and we want to get our workouts finished as quickly as possible, if only in the interest of time management. But getting your muscles warmed up (you need some light "warm-up" exercises before stretching out your muscles) at the beginning of your workout helps you to avoid injuries. It also helps get the blood flow started, which in turn makes for a better workout. Stretching after your workout helps to maintain flexibility and speeds muscle recovery.

2. *Cardiovascular exercise.* This kind of exercise gets the heart pumping, the blood flowing, and the lungs working. Cardiovascular exercise should be part of every man's workout routine. This is how you give your lungs and heart a good workout and how you burn fat or maintain your present weight.

One of the great things about cardiovascular exercise is that you don't have to pay for a membership at the local gym or buy expensive equipment to get it. You can get your heart rate up through simple exercises like walking or jogging.

3. *Resistance exercise.* By resistance exercise, I mean lifting weights with dumbbells, "free weights," or using your own body weight to strengthen your muscles. Does resistance exercise bring up your testosterone levels? Some researchers believe this kind of exercise elevates a man's testosterone level only temporarily—while he's working out—but that it drops again or levels out soon after the workout concludes. Others believe that over the long term, it can help increase the overall level of serum testosterone. Make sure you learn how to perform resistance exercise with the proper technique by having a fitness expert or trainer show you how.

Many men find it easier to get the exercise they need when a friend or partner offers to join them. It's not only a great way for couples to get in shape, it also can become a fun time for enjoying each other.

Watch What You Eat

A healthy, testosterone-maintaining or boosting diet should include a good balance of proteins, fats, and carbohydrates. The key word here is *balance*. Your whole body, including the systems that produce testosterone, requires you to consume the right amounts of proteins, fats (forget the low-fat diets), and carbs.

Consider a few things to focus on in relation to healthy testosterone levels:

Eat your fruits and vegetables. That's not just good advice from Mom, it's also a key to keeping your testosterone levels where they need to be. Eat lots of veggies, especially green, leafy ones and cruciferous vegetables like broccoli, cauliflower, kale, Swiss chard, Brussels sprouts, and cabbage. The fresher the better!

Cut out the junk food. In the classic comic strip "Calvin and Hobbes," a little boy named Calvin started his day with a "nutritious" breakfast of Chocolate-Covered Sugar Bombs. Diet-wise, it was probably all downhill for Calvin after that!

We Americans consume a staggering amount of junk food (the term is only half right), and it's only a matter of time before we suffer the negative health effects that such a diet will bring our way. Heavily refined, high-carbohydrate foods like cookies, candies, ice cream, and many others offer little in the way of real nutrition, and they can cause a spike in your blood sugar, which causes elevated levels of insulin and cortisol, both of which can lower testosterone production.

Here's my advice: If it has a funny brand name and contains lots of sugar and white flour, *don't eat it!*

Eat healthy fats. Omega 3 fatty acids (found in fish and flaxseed) and saturated fats are vital for testosterone production. Testosterone comes from cholesterol, and when the body lacks cholesterol, testosterone levels suffer. So don't let the word *fat* scare you away from consuming it; just make sure it's the right kind of fat.

Get your zinc. You've probably heard stories about how eating raw oysters are a sure ticket to a strong libido. The stories have an element of truth. Zinc is essential to the production of testosterone, which gives a man his sex drive. Oysters have more zinc per serving than any other food; but if you don't like oysters, then consider red meat and poultry, which also contain good amounts of zinc. Other zinc-providing foods include beans, nuts, some seafoods (crab and lobster, for example), whole grains, and dairy products.

Use a quality multi-vitamin supplement. Ideally, we shouldn't have to use vitamin supplements, but making sure we get the vitamins and minerals we need can be a real challenge. So it doesn't hurt to take *quality* supplements that include vitamins A (which decreases the production of estrogen in the testicles), E (stimulates production of sex hormones), C (enhances pituitary function, which can help raise testosterone levels), and B6 (helps decrease the secretion of prolactin), as well as a good daily dosage of zinc—all of which help in testosterone production. To reduce the body's estrogen level, I recommend a 50 milligram dosage of zinc, three days a week.

Testosterone-Boosting Foods

Meats & Fish

Oysters
Poultry
Red Meat
Salmon

Fruits and Vegetables

Apples
Asparagus
Avocadoes
Bananas
Blackberries
Blueberries
Broccoli
Brussels Sprouts
Cabbage
Cantaloupe
Carrots
Cauliflower
Citrus fruits
Figs

Kale
Mangoes
Papaya
Pineapple
Raspberries
Red Peppers
Spinach
Swiss Chard
Tomatoes

Grains

Brown rice

Dairy

Cheese
Cottage Cheese
Milk
Yogurt

Other

Almonds
Beans

Eggs
Fish Oil
Olive Oil
Peanuts
Pine Nuts
Pumpkin Seeds
Walnuts

A Final Word on Avoiding Low T Risk Factors

While you can't eliminate *all* risk factors for Low T, you can minimize your risk by making healthy lifestyle choices. And when you make decisions that help your body's production of testosterone, your whole body functions better. Regardless of your current testosterone level, recognize that none of the things I've suggested in this chapter will help you do anything but avoid Low T or recover from Low T.

And isn't that the point?

CHAPTER NINE

A Wonder Drug ... or Just Good Medicine?

The Benefits and Risks of Testosterone Replacement Therapy

In the nineteenth and early twentieth centuries, hucksters often traveled from town to town by horse and wagon, peddling a variety of "miracle elixirs." They claimed these magical potions had the power to cure any disease, prolong life, and help the consumer to feel better.

Of course, the elixir had no power to cure anything—except, perhaps, the seller's net worth—and the only reason some buyers felt better after using it was that they *believed* they would. These traveling medicine shows created a public wary of "snake oil," a term associated with utterly worthless "medicinal" potions and mixtures.

While I would never suggest that testosterone is some kind of wonder drug or magic elixir that will cure everything that ails you, there is no doubt that testosterone deficient men can receive several benefits from testosterone replacement therapy. We were meant to thrive on a certain level of testosterone, and maintaining that level is the key.

We've already seen how men who receive TRT often enjoy improved sexual desire and performance, as well as an improved mood and overall outlook. Many men who suffer from Low T have found that they just feel better and enjoy life more once they've begun TRT and given the therapy time to do its work.

Before we discuss in detail the benefits of testosterone therapy for men who suffer from Low T, consider the following short list of such benefits:

- Improved sexual function (libido and erections)
- Increased level of energy
- Increased lean muscle mass
- Decreased fat mass
- Increased muscle strength
- Increased bone density
- Correction of anemia
- Improved insulin sensitivity and blood glucose control in men with metabolic syndrome or type 2 diabetes

Men with Low T who begin a doctor-approved regiment of TRT have good reason for optimism, even if they're well along in years! Now let's take a closer look at some of the known (or suspected) benefits of TRT.

The Sexual Benefits

As we've seen, testosterone plays a vital role in a man's sexuality. Without getting too technical, I'll explain how it affects the parts of the brain that give a man his sex drive and the ability to perform sexually (in other words, to have an erection). It also has a huge effect on the male sex organs—the penis, the testicles, the prostate, and the seminal vesicles.

All of the organs just listed must work efficiently together for the man to have normal, pleasurable sexual experiences. And when one of them malfunctions—due to Low Testosterone or other medical or emotional/relational problems—sexual dysfunction occurs in the form of low libido, erectile dysfunction, and other difficulties.

When a man in an otherwise healthy, loving relationship either becomes disinterested in sex or is unable to perform, Low Testosterone is often the culprit. For many men, testosterone replacement therapy is the ticket back to a high quality sex life.

Increased Libido

Several theories try to explain how testosterone produces the sex drive in men. Some things we know for certain. For example, we know that testosterone works on the parts of the brain that give the man his sex drive. We also know that it's perfectly normal for a man's sex drive to slowly and steadily decline from its peak in his teens and 20s.

Many factors can affect a man's sex drive. Men who feel "stressed out" at work or at home may see a decreased sex drive. Also, fatigue due to overwork or lack of sleep can cause noticeable declines in a man's sex drive, at least over the short term. Depression and other medical problems can also sap a man's hunger for sex. Usually, however, once he deals with the stress or fatigue or the depression or other medical issues, his libido returns to normal. When a man's sex drive drops to below normal (and what's "normal" varies from man to man; some maintain a very high sex drive into middle age and beyond, while others have a much lower libido, even in their twenties) over a longer period of time, however, it may signal Low Testosterone.

Not all men who have Low Testosterone levels also have low libidos. Some maintain normal libidos, while some see only a slight drop in their sex drives. Nearly every reputable study I've seen, however, shows that the percentages of men with low libido are much higher for men with Low T than with those with normal testosterone levels.

In my practice (as well as in my personal experience), I've seen TRT bring the patient's sex drive back to normal. Yet it doesn't work like an erectile dysfunction drug. As you begin your TRT program, remind yourself and your partner to be patient, because it will take time for the full effects of the testosterone to kick in. How long varies from patient to patient. Some men see noticeable improvements relatively quickly; others have to be more patient. In general, most patients who undergo TRT should see an increase in their libidos in three or four weeks, with the full effect taking place in about three months.

Some words of caution here: Testosterone therapy won't help a man regain his desire for his partner if the problem has its roots in a relational or emotional difficulty. Certainly, a man who suffers from Low T and is in a dysfunctional or troubled relationship will regain his libido—but his relationship problems will remain. In fact, restoring a man's libido through TRT when his relationship is in trouble may create *other* problems, because he may then look elsewhere to put his newly restored libido to the test. In cases like these, both the testosterone deficiency *and* the problems within the relationship need to be addressed, both directly and simultaneously.

Also, erectile dysfunction drugs like Viagra, Levitra, and Cialis usually don't do much to increase a man's libido. If the loss of libido is due to erectile dysfunction, then they may help. But it is quite possible for a man with low libido to attain rock-hard erections but have little or no interest in doing anything sexual with them.

Improved Erections

The first benefit that men who begin testosterone therapy hope to enjoy is an increase in libido—the *desire* to have sex. The second benefit is an improvement in his erections—the *ability* to perform sexually.

A man's penis is very much like a balloon—okay, a balloon with a very complicated process of "inflation." An erection occurs when an extra flow of blood fills two spongy, erectile bodies inside the shaft of the penis (the corpus cavernosum). It sounds simple, doesn't it? But how this all comes about is an amazing, complex chain of events involving the brain, the nervous system, hormones (such as testosterone), and blood vessels.

It all starts with messages from the brain. A man receives some kind of sexual stimulation—a thought, a touch, something he sees or hears, or any combination of these things—and the brain says, "Hey, buddy! Woo-hoo!" The erection begins when the brain sends messages down the spinal cord to the many blood vessels and tissues involved in an erection. These messages cause the smooth muscles in the blood vessel walls of the corpus cavernosum to relax, allowing more blood to flow through the vessels and fill the corpus cavernosum. At the same moment, the veins that carry blood away from the penis get shut down, which causes an increase in blood pressure in the penis. The blood trapped within the corpus cavernosum causes the penis to become hard and erect.

Scientists aren't exactly sure what specific role testosterone plays in a man's erectile health, but we do know that one of the major symptoms of Low T is erectile dysfunction. A lot of Low T patients report improvement in ED symptoms when they begin therapy. These men also begin to have morning erections again, which is the body's way of keeping the hydraulic system well maintained.

Like low libido, several factors can affect a man's ability to achieve and maintain an erection firm enough to engage in sexual intercourse. High blood pressure, diabetes, injury to the penis, and stress are just a few of the culprits. Cigarette smoking, excessive alcohol use, and some prescription and over-the-counter drugs certainly don't help, either.

And where does testosterone replacement therapy fit in? Until very recently—within the last decade and a half or so—the medical community wasn't at all sure that TRT had any direct effect on improving erectile dysfunction. In fact, some authorities declared that it had been overprescribed as a treatment for ED, and that it had little or no effect on the condition. Still others said it had a placebo effect; the patient *believed* the testosterone would improve his erections, and as a result, he actually had better erections.

I'm happy to report that the most up-to-date studies, as well as the observations of many physicians, myself included, have shown that TRT can *directly* affect many patients' ability to achieve erections satisfactory for sexual intercourse. Medical science has learned that testosterone affects not just the sexual centers of the brain, but also the vascular structures of the penis itself, as well as other parts of the body that play parts in the process of an erection. So it only makes sense that TRT can, at least for some patients, be an effective part of treating Low T-related erectile dysfunction.

Testosterone replacement therapy has even been shown to improve erections in men who have tried the standard erectile dysfunction drugs—sometimes in larger-than-usual doses—without much success. Furthermore, even if the TRT doesn't give the patient firm enough erections, it can help give drugs like Viagra, Levitra, and Cialis that extra "push" to make them effective in men who had enjoyed little success with them before.

Some things about TRT have a clear effect on a man's ability to perform sexually. First, it improves the patient's libido; and although a higher libido doesn't always equal better erections, an increased "drive" can certainly have an effect on the patient's ability to achieve a satisfactory erection. Second, TRT can improve the patient's outlook and sense of well-being (more on that later), which can improve his feelings of virility and masculinity. A man who feels like a man is more likely to perform better sexually.

The bottom line is this: We know that TRT can help men with erectile problems. The medical evidence proves it, and I've seen it in my own practice.

Decreased Fat/Increased Lean Muscle Mass

The word "testosterone" received a bad rap a few decades back when the public became aware that many high-profile athletes had turned to anabolic steroids—as we've seen, these are essentially synthetic forms of the natural hormone testosterone—in order to "gain an edge." Sports fans, as well as those involved in athletics at various levels, responded to this unscrupulous practice by branding those who used these dangerous drugs as "cheaters." Keep in mind, though, that these athletes who abused testosterone were using *10 to 100 times* the safe dose.

And why did so many athletes over the past few decades ignore the risks and give into the temptation to use anabolic steroids? It's simple: They work!

The same holds true for doctor-prescribed testosterone replacement therapy—but without the dangerous side effects. When used properly, TRT can have amazingly positive effects on the patient's body composition.

One symptom of Low T is an increase in body fat, especially around the midsection, and a decrease in lean muscle mass. That is largely because one of testosterone's many functions is to aid the body in developing larger, stronger muscles. This explains why young boys begin to develop physically around puberty and why, all things being equal, women generally don't develop the same size or strength of muscles as men.

For men whose bodies have undergone the changes associated with Low T—the reduction of muscle mass and the associated loss of physical strength, as well as the "spare tire" around the midsection—TRT has been shown to increase lean muscle mass while at the same time decreasing fat mass. Some studies have shown that testosterone aids in fat loss in several important ways. First, it seems to reduce fat storage by blocking an enzyme called lipoprotein lipase, which aids fat cells in absorbing more fat. Testosterone also has been shown to aid the body in burning excess fat.

Testosterone in higher levels has two other important effects on muscle mass: It increases the size and strength of muscle cells the patient already has, and in a process called "recruitment," it helps the body convert nearby cells into muscle cells.

In an example of how TRT affects the patient's body in ways you might not expect, many men who receive the treatment actually find that they *gain* weight, even though they lose body fat. This depends, of course, on the amount of excess fat the patient carried in the first place; but the men who gain weight after beginning TRT tend to gain that weight simply because lean muscle weighs more than fat.

One other point to consider is that the more muscle you have, the more energy it takes to maintain that muscle. This causes an increase in your body's metabolic rate, which means you burn more calories while doing absolutely nothing with this new added muscle.

Increased Bone Density

One treatment for prostate cancer radically lowers the patient's testosterone level (see chapter 10). That's because testosterone can speed the progression of the disease (though, as you'll read later, no evidence suggests that TRT increases the risk of prostate cancer). One of the side effects of this testosterone-lowering treatment is decreased bone density and an increased risk of fractures.

Low Testosterone levels can drastically increase a man's risk of developing osteoporosis (a thinning of the bones), a disease found mostly in women. That condition weakens the bones, leaving the patient vulnerable to fractures of the hip and other areas due to relatively minor injuries. Over the past few decades, study after study has shown conclusively that, over time—maybe up to three years—TRT can drastically improve bone density in patients with Low T. Of course, improvements in bone density under *any* treatment for thinning bones will take just as long as TRT.

Improved Mood and Energy Levels

For the partner of a man whose testosterone levels have dipped, probably the most noticeable symptoms of Low T (other than a decreased interest in sex) are the changes in mood and energy levels. She notices that he just isn't the same man he used to be, that he seems more moody and less energetic than before. Even more disturbingly, perhaps, he appears to prefer solitude more than he once did.

In fact, Low Testosterone often makes a man feel crummy. He feels tired all the time, he can't think straight, and he finds himself getting agitated at things he might not even have noticed before. He wants to be alone more than previously, and when he gets alone he feels tired, out of energy, and just wants to sleep. Unfortunately, no amount of rest is enough for the man suffering from Low T.

The good news for such men is that TRT has been shown to improve both mood and energy levels, sometimes shortly after treatment starts. Whereas before treatment the Low T sufferer seemed somber and negative, he now has a better outlook on life and begins enjoying the things that previously brought him pleasure. His energy level returns to normal and he regains his self-confidence.

In short, he gets his mojo back!

Again, however, we shouldn't see testosterone as some kind of miraculous "mood drug." A man who was temperamental, moody, and surly *before* his testosterone levels dropped will undoubtedly be the same temperamental, moody, surly man he was after he begins receiving TRT. The only difference will be that he will be back to normal— normal for *him*.

Overcoming Depression

Testosterone treatment has been shown to help men who have spiraled into depression due to the effects of Low T.

The idea that testosterone treatment can help the Low T sufferer overcome bouts of depression goes back to the 1920s, when doctors attempted to treat lethargic men with a serum made of ground-up animal testicles. Though this serum probably had little real affect, other than as a placebo, doctors believed that it contained the essence of male virility and would therefore help listless men get back to normal. Later, in the

'40s and '50s, doctors began prescribing injections of actual testosterone as a treatment for depression.

Recent studies have proven that the doctors who prescribed testosterone to treat depression in men got some things right. One recent study examined the effects of testosterone gel on a group of men diagnosed with clinical depression, but who had not responded to antidepressants. Half of these men had unusually Low Testosterone levels, and after using testosterone gel for eight weeks, they reported significant improvements in their mood, less anxiety, and that they slept better than men in the same study who had been treated with a placebo gel. I believe every man being treated for depression should have his testosterone checked prior to starting any antidepressant medications.

Correction of Anemia

Anemia is a common blood disorder in which the patient suffers a decrease in red blood cells or a decrease in the ability of the red blood cells to transport oxygen from the lungs to the body's tissues and organs.

Since Low Testosterone levels can help to cause anemia, TRT can keep the red blood cell count where it needs to be and so prevent anemia from developing. TRT also can correct anemia in testosterone deficient patients who already have developed the disorder.

Possible Lowered Cholesterol Levels

The word "cholesterol" can strike fear into the hearts of those concerned about their health. And such concern is justified, because elevated levels of cholesterol put people at higher risk for cardiovascular disease.

Understand, however, that there are two main types of cholesterol. First is the high-density lipoprotein (HDL), known as "good" cholesterol because it helps protect against hardening of the arteries and heart disease. Second is the "bad" cholesterol, low density lipoprotein (LDL), which at higher levels dramatically increases the chances for heart disease.

At one time, doctors believed that higher levels of testosterone could raise cholesterol levels; but like many other beliefs about testosterone, that opinion has changed. Now, due to the findings of several studies, the medical community believes that a healthy level of testosterone may actually *lower* total cholesterol levels (or that it has no effect at all on cholesterol).

Possible Improvement in Cardiovascular Health

Many of the *possible* benefits of TRT have to be placed in the "wait and see" category. Research on the benefits of testosterone remains a work in progress, but some evidence suggests that TRT may improve a man's cardiovascular health and therefore lower his risk of developing cardiovascular disease. Some relatively new evidence even suggests that testosterone may help protect against atherosclerosis (hardening of the arteries) and arterial clogging.

Possible Improvements in Low T Diabetics

While it is not known whether Low T helps to cause diabetes, or whether diabetes helps to cause Low T (or if both are true), some medical evidence suggests that TRT may benefit men at high risk for diabetes. It appears that testosterone therapy may have a positive effect on risk factors for diabetes such as obesity, low insulin sensitivity, glucose control, and blood lipid profiles—all of which are common in men with Low Testosterone. Diabetic patients who have started TRT notice that controlling their blood sugar becomes much easier.

Possible Risks of TRT

Testosterone replacement therapy is a very safe option for testosterone-deficient men who want to enjoy the benefits of returning their testosterone levels to normal. Yet it is not without *some* health risks. Still, I believe that, for most people, the benefits appear to far outweigh the risks.

The risks and side effects range from uncommon to extremely rare. Before you and your partner decide to start TRT, make sure that you talk to your doctor about the risk factors and what you can do to lessen them. Consider a few things you and your doctor should look for:

- *BPH (Benign Prostatic Hyperplasia).* TRT *may* cause enlargement of the prostate in some men, also known as BPH. This is not the same as prostate cancer, though some connection exists between the two (we'll discuss testosterone and prostate cancer more in chapter 10). BPH is a very common condition in older men. An enlarged prostate can be uncomfortable and can cause problems with urination.

- *Gynecomastia (male breast growth).* This rare side effect of TRT occurs when the body converts testosterone into estrogen. This condition does not endanger a man's health, but it can feel uncomfortable (those affected commonly report tenderness in the nipple area). The condition can be reversed by stopping TRT or by use of a medication called anastrozole (Arimidex). Another option is surgical removal of the breast tissue.

- *Fluid Retention/Generalized Edema.* This very uncommon (and usually temporary) side effect of TRT involves localized swelling in various parts of the body, such as the ankles. Men with congestive heart failure are at a higher risk of developing this problem.

- *Polycythemia (High Red Blood Cell Count).* Also known as erythrocytosis, this condition can cause the blood to become too thick, possibly leading to clogged arteries, which could result in a stroke or heart attack. Men on TRT can have an increase in their volume of red blood cells (the hematocrit) and in their hemoglobin. TRT presents a very real risk of polycythemia, so men receiving TRT should have their hematocrit or hemoglobin checked regularly—once or twice during the first year, and annually after that. The condition can be corrected by stopping TRT or by adjusting dosages. The patient also can have blood drawn (a procedure called therapeutic phlebotomy) and discarded or donated to a blood bank.

- *Exacerbation of Sleep Apnea.* In this potentially dangerous condition, someone stops breathing for short periods during sleep. TRT has been known to worsen this problem, though instances are uncommon.
- *Acne.* In some individuals, TRT can increase the production of oil from glands in the skin, leading to acne.
- *Weight Gain.* This may be due to fluid retention in the TRT patient, or due to replacement of fatty tissue with lean muscle tissue.
- *Rash.* Some patients using testosterone patches or gels have been known to develop localized rashes.
- *Shrinkage of the testicles.* This condition, known as "testicular atrophy," occurs in a small number of TRT patients.
- *Liver Damage.* Liver damage may occur in men who use oral testosterone replacement therapy, a treatment option that I strongly discourage. The Food and Drug Administration requires all testosterone products to include on their labels the danger of liver damage. Other forms of testosterone replacement therapy (injections, patches, or creams/gels) present *no* known risk of liver problems.
- *High Blood Pressure.* Rare instances have been reported of increased blood pressure in TRT patients. This may be due to instances of fluid retention associated with TRT. At the same time, however, I have noticed many patients who actually lower their blood pressure after starting TRT.
- *Infertility.* Testosterone therapy can lower sperm counts in some men, often to zero or near zero. For this reason, medical researchers are currently studying the possible use of testosterone

for male birth control. Low or non-existent sperm counts due to TRT pose no additional health risks, but men who wish to father children should discuss this issue with their physician before going on TRT.

Based on recent research, I have begun using a drug called Clomid (Clomiphene)—originally developed as an ovarian stimulant for women—to help the testicles produce more testosterone and increase a man's sperm count. I use it with younger patients with Low T who still want to have children; I have seen some encouraging results with these men in as little as a month. The most recent research shows that Clomid may work in older men, as well.

- *Moodiness/Irritability.* Some men on TRT have reported changes in their moods, that they feel more moody and temperamental than before. In the vast majority of cases, however, TRT has been found to stabilize patients' moods.

Should You Seek Treatment?

As you consider the risks of TRT, remember that these are *possible* side effects. *None* of them are the norm; in fact, many are quite rare. I don't include them in this chapter to scare you away from pursuing TRT, but to make you aware of the potential risks so that you can be ready to deal with them if you encounter them in your own TRT experience.

Second, let me emphasize that TRT is a very safe medical treatment, so long as certain health factors are monitored during the early stages of treatment. That monitoring should include a prostate-specific antigen (PSA) at 6 months after beginning treatment, as well as yearly with a digital rectal exam (DRE), just to rule out problems with the prostate gland. A 6 month and yearly hematocrit check (to rule out problems with the red blood cell count) is also needed.

The bottom line?

Testosterone replacement therapy, so long as a reliable health care professional monitors it, is very safe and carries minimal risk of side effects. An otherwise healthy man with Low T likely will find great benefit and very little risk in beginning a regimen of TRT.

CHAPTER TEN

What about Prostate Cancer?

Testosterone Replacement Therapy and the Prostate Gland

"**D**octor, this testosterone replacement therapy sounds just like what my husband needs. It might make him feel better and get him back to being the man I've always known and loved. But I have one fear—I've heard that it can cause prostate cancer. I'd rather have him stay the way he is right now, than to feel better for a while and then get cancer."

While I can't speak for every urologist, I'm always glad when one of my patients or his partner brings up what they think they know or have heard about the connection between testosterone replacement therapy and prostate cancer. I want my patients to have all the information available to them before they decide that testosterone replacement therapy is for them; but more than that, I want them to fully understand the real connections between the "Big C" and TRT.

Before we get into the real meat of this chapter, I need to say that there absolutely *are* links between testosterone and prostate cancer. But before I tell the story of how the medical community once believed that

TRT increases the risk of prostate cancer, I'll let you know up front that, despite what you may have heard, *testosterone replacement therapy does not cause prostate cancer*. In fact, it doesn't even increase the risk of this disease—despite the almost universal belief a few years ago that TRT posed an increased risk of prostate cancer. In those days, men considering testosterone replacement, and their doctors, believed they had to weigh the well-documented benefits of TRT against what they believed to be a real and serious increase in the risk for prostate cancer.

And where did the long-held position get started? From a doctor who won the Nobel Prize for his research! But before we get to that story, let's take a quick look at what the prostate is and what it does.

Important Things to Know about the Prostate

What many people know about the prostate gland is limited to what they see on television commercials. They know it can become inflamed and enlarged, and that it causes a man trouble when it does so.

But what, actually, does the prostate gland *do*?

A healthy prostate is a walnut-sized gland located at the base of the bladder in men. It surrounds the urethra, the tube-like organ that goes from the bladder and through the end of the penis. It provides lubricant for sexual intercourse (though it supplies relatively little), which it secretes into the urethra. The fluid excreted through the prostate also carries sperm during ejaculation.

Common Diseases of the Prostate

Three main disorders affect the prostate: inflammation (also called prostatitis), benign growth (also known as benign prostatic hyperplasia, or BPH, a possible side effect of TRT for some men), and cancer. The most common of the three is BPH, which affects around 50 percent of men aged 60 and older and about 90 percent of men who reach 85 years of age. The word *hyperplasia* refers to an abnormal increase in the number of cells. The best-known symptom of BPH is frequent urination, getting up frequently at night to urinate, hesitancy at the start of urination, and reduced force in the urinary stream.

BPH is not caused by sexual activity, or the lack of it, and developing BPH does not increase the odds of developing prostate cancer. It is a treatable condition, both with medication and with surgery.

Prostate cancer is the most commonly diagnosed malignancy in men in the US (around 200,000 diagnoses yearly) and the second-leading cause of deaths in American men (after lung cancer), killing around 30,000 men a year. The risk of prostate cancer increases with age, and cases of the disease in men under 50 are unusual. Age and genetics (some families seem to have a history of prostate cancer) are the most important risk factors for prostate cancer. Sexual activity, or lack of it, are not risk factors for this disease.

On a positive note, a diagnosis of prostate cancer usually carries with it a good prognosis. Improvements in early detection and in treatment have made prostate cancer a very survivable disease. In fact, prostate cancer deaths have been declining in the US for the past several years. And even before the development of superior prostate cancer detection and treatment, only about one in seven men diagnosed with the disease actually died from it. That is largely because prostate cancer is usually a very slow-growing malignancy and because most men diagnosed with the disease were older individuals who later died of other causes.

This brief history brings us back to the story of how testosterone treatment was once falsely labeled as a risk factor for prostate cancer.

Testosterone Research Gone to the Dogs

In his excellent book *Testosterone for Life*, Dr. Abraham Morgentaler tells the story of how the medical community came to what seemed an indisputable fact: Testosterone therapy increases the risk of prostate cancer.

It all started way back in the 1940s—the dark ages, it seems, when it comes to testosterone research—when Charles B. Huggins

(1901–97), an esteemed urologist at the University of Chicago, began using dogs (that's right, dogs!) in his research. At first, Huggins was interested in researching benign prostatic hyperplasia (BPH), which causes uncomfortable enlargement of the prostate and is very common in older men.

Huggins knew one interesting fact about dogs: They are the only animal on earth, other than human beings, known to commonly develop problems with the prostate. From the turn of the century up to that time, one of the treatments for severe cases of BPH was castration—a radical step that most men, as you might imagine, felt extremely reluctant to take.

Huggins noted that castration worked in shrinking the swollen prostates of dogs. But he also noted that microscopic spots in some of these dogs' prostates were identical to those of human prostate cancer. Not only that, he noticed that castration, which cut off the animals' supply of testosterone, also caused these areas to clear up. He could find no more evidence of canine prostate cancer.

Huggins and his associates began to apply what they'd seen in their research on canines to humans. They worked with a group of men suffering from prostate cancer, which already had spread to their bones. They lowered the men's testosterone levels either by removing their testicles or by administering doses of estrogen. Eventually, they concluded that reducing testosterone levels caused these men's prostate cancers to shrink—and that raising their testosterone levels caused the cancer to grow more rapidly.

An Incomplete Truth

The first part of Huggins's conclusion represented an important discovery, because until then, medical science had no treatment for prostate cancer. Since that time, prostate cancers have been treated successfully by lowering testosterone levels, either through castration or through estrogen treatments.

(In the 1980s, a new treatment for lowering testosterone was developed, eliminating the need for castration, which even men suffering from prostate cancer didn't care for, or for dosages of estrogen, which can cause heart attacks and blood clots in men. This medication, called LHRH [luteinizing hormone-releasing hormone] Agonists, is now the standard way to lower testosterone levels in men with prostate cancer.)

The second part of Huggins's conclusion about the relationship between testosterone and prostate cancer led the medical community to see a cause/effect relationship between the two. They believed that increasing a man's testosterone levels increased his risk of developing prostate cancer. This meant testosterone-deficient men and their doctors faced a dilemma: either leave the testosterone deficiency untreated and suffer the very real symptoms and effects of Low T, or treat the testosterone deficiency and face the possibility of developing prostate cancer.

Since that time, however, many reliable studies—including Morgentaler's—have concluded that raising a man's testosterone levels through TRT absolutely does *not* put him at higher risk for prostate cancer. What's more, several studies have shown that *low* testosterone levels may put men at a higher risk for developing prostate cancer.

Maybe the death knell for the idea that high testosterone puts a man at higher risk for prostate cancer sounded in 2008, when a study published in the *Journal of the National Cancer Institute* concluded that high testosterone does not increase the risk of prostate cancer. In this study, authors of eighteen separate studies pooled their data concerning the relationship between high testosterone and prostate cancer. The study included more than 3,000 men with prostate cancer and 6,000 without. Absolutely *no* connection was found between prostate cancer and any of the hormones studied, including testosterone.

While testosterone treatment does not and cannot cause new cancers to develop, however, many studies have shown that it can cause already existing cancer—cancer in its earliest development—to grow and develop. In other words, the testosterone didn't *cause* the cancer, it only "fertilized" it, as one expert on the subject has written, and caused it to grow—and to be diagnosed earlier than it otherwise would have been. Yet even here, Morgentaler has discovered that increasing the amounts of testosterone in a man's system do not trigger cancer growth; the cancer is already saturated with testosterone, and more testosterone neither increases the growth of the cancer nor triggers it to begin growing.

Think of it like this. Suppose a young reporter working for his hometown newspaper got wind of some serious financial malfeasance on the part of some of local elected officials, maybe even the mayor himself. Maybe someone tipped him off, or maybe he noticed some inconsistencies in some records he routinely examined; it really doesn't matter how he found out. After digging around and looking at the town's financial records, the reporter and his editor became convinced that improprieties indeed had taken place. The next day, a front page story exposed the shenanigans. So what before had been some local officials secretly dipping into the city till, became a full-blown public scandal.

Would anyone but the most rabid partisan suggest that this ambitious, young reporter "caused" the chicanery going on at City Hall? Of course not! The reporter didn't *cause* anything; he simply exposed to the public what already was going on. And once the deeds were brought to light, heads rolled.

Something very much like this can happen when a man with previously undetected prostate cancer begins TRT: The testosterone doesn't cause the cancer, it only exposes what was already going on in his body, and so gives him and his doctors a chance to correct the situation before it can grow any worse.

The Facts Don't Lie

The great American humorist and author Mark Twain once said, "A lie can travel halfway around the world while the truth is putting on its shoes." That is certainly true of the idea that testosterone therapy can cause cancer—or at least, that it can increase the risk of developing the disease.

Stop and think about it for a moment. At what time in a man's life is his testosterone level the highest? Clearly, it reaches its highest levels during his teens and twenties. And when is it lowest? When he gets older, normally starting in his forties and decreasing incrementally the older he gets. So if high levels of testosterone really caused prostate cancer, then wouldn't it make sense that it would be more common among younger men? And yet it isn't.

Moreover, the most reliable medical research available today demonstrates beyond a doubt that the older the man is *and* the lower his testosterone levels are, the higher his risk for developing cancer. There are a few other risk factors for prostate cancer, such as diet and ethnicity, but age and testosterone levels, as connected as they almost always are, are two of the main culprits.

Finally, there's the medical evidence gleaned from many studies proving that TRT does not increase a man's risk of prostate cancer. In some of these studies, cancer incidences were compared between groups of men on testosterone therapy and the general male population. And guess what? The percentages of men in each group who, at some point, were diagnosed with prostate cancer were identical.

In fact, there is *no* credible evidence that TRT increases the risk of prostate cancer. The evidence actually points overwhelmingly in the opposite direction: It is *lower* testosterone levels in men that increases the risk of prostate cancer, not higher ones.

But old ideas can die slow and painful deaths, even in the medical community. Many medical professionals still fear that TRT can lead to higher risks of prostate cancer. (Just type the phrases "prostate cancer" and "testosterone treatment" into your web browser, and you'll see what I mean.)

So if you and your partner are considering treatment for Low T, please put out of your minds the idea that it could cause prostate cancer. If you're concerned about early stage prostate cancer, then get tested. That will not only reassure you about the risks of TRT, it will also (at worst) reveal a very treatable medical condition.

TRT and Prostate Cancer:
The *Real* Cause for Concern

Dr. Huggins's discovery that reducing testosterone levels—in dogs and men alike—can cause prostate cancer to shrink is still widely accepted in the medical community today. His second conclusion that higher levels of testosterone can actually "feed" hungry prostate cancer cells and cause it to progress more rapidly is still being determined.

One of the most important parts of my patients' medical profile I have to check before I even think of prescribing TRT is whether he has prostate cancer. It takes a couple of steps to diagnose prostate cancer. If the patient demonstrates certain symptoms (see sidebar) or if screening tests such as the prostate-specific antigen (PSA) blood test and/or digital rectal exam (DRE) point to the possibility of cancer, the doctor will then do a prostate biopsy to find out for sure if the patient has the disease.

Prostate Cancer Symptoms

In its early stages, prostate cancer may not cause any noticeable signs or symptoms; but in its more advanced stages, it may cause the following:

- Difficulty urinating
- Decreased force in the stream of urine

- Blood in the urine
- Blood in the semen
- Swelling in the legs
- Discomfort in the pelvic area
- Bone pain

Please be aware that these symptoms could also point to other problems with the prostate, such as BPH. The only way to know for sure if the symptoms are due to prostate cancer is to see your doctor for a diagnosis.

A biopsy is a simple, relatively painless procedure that involves taking a sample of body tissue (in this case, from the prostate gland) and examining it under a microscope to look for cancer cells.

What About After the Cancer Is Gone?

The bad news nationally is that some 200,000 American men will be diagnosed with prostate cancer this year, and probably every year after. The good news, however, is that a good majority of those men will survive and that many of the survivors will be treated, fully recover, and go on to live healthy, cancer-free lives.

But is there more good news? Specifically, what about the prostate cancer survivor who happens to suffer from Low T? He's already heard that terrifying announcement, "You have cancer," but he's also gone through the treatments and has been given a completely clean bill of health—at least in regard to prostate cancer.

After a scare like that, it only makes sense that a man would want to do everything he could to squeeze everything he can out of the days he has remaining on this earth (and he's grateful there appear to be many more!). So maybe, just maybe, he's thinking about getting treated for Low T.

But is it safe?

The short, and admittedly not very satisfying, answer to that important question is that we just don't know yet. We don't know the risks, and we don't know the percentages of men previously diagnosed and treated for prostate cancer who might relapse if they were to raise their testosterone levels through TRT.

I wish I could say that giving TRT to a man who has fully recovered from prostate cancer is completely safe, with little to no chance that the treatment could cause the cancer to reappear. But I don't want to downplay the possible risks of introducing new testosterone into the body of a prostate cancer survivor.

For the past six-plus decades, the prevailing position within the medical community was that TRT presented too much of a risk of "awakening" dormant prostate cancer cells and causing a recurrence of the disease. But seeds of change in that position have been planted, and it's possible that future research will demonstrate that treating prostate cancer survivors with testosterone is no more risky than treating anyone else.

In *Testosterone for Life*, Dr. Morgentaler stated that a number of doctors had told him that they had occasionally treated patients with testosterone "despite the fact that they'd been treated for prostate cancer in the past." He also referred to an article by Drs. Joel Kaufman and James Graydon, the first physicians to publish their experiences with treating prostate cancer survivors with testosterone. In the article, which appeared in the *Journal of Urology* in 2004, Kaufman and Graydon recounted their experiences in treating seven men with TRT after they had undergone radical prostatectomy as their treatment for prostate cancer. The longest follow-up was twelve years, and all seven remained cancer free.

Not long after the publication of Kaufman and Graydon's article, another paper, this one by a group from Case Western Reserve University School of Medicine, described similar results in ten men with an average follow-up of about nineteen months. Still another group, one from

Baylor College of Medicine, reported the same results in twenty-one prostate cancer survivors.

That's a total of 38 men—and without a single recurrence of prostate cancer.

Morgentaler cites another experience, published by Dr. Michael Sarosdy, who recorded and reported the results of TRT in a group of thirty-one men who had received a different kind of prostate cancer treatment: Radioactive seeds, called brachytherapy, a form of treatment that does not involve surgical removal of the prostate. In theory, since each of these men still had their prostate glands, each of them faced the possibility that some residue of the cancer might still lie dormant in their prostates and that the testosterone might "awaken" them. After an average follow-up of five years, however, not one of the men had *any* evidence of recurrence of prostate cancer.

Morgentaler admits that the total number of men treated in these reports is much too small for anyone to take the definitive position that TRT is absolutely safe for men who have had prostate cancer, but who now are cancer-free. But he also points out that they provide evidence that TRT does not appear to be associated with a risk of the recurrence of prostate cancer, at least over the first several years of treatment.

In my practice I have a small group of men who have Low T and are on TRT, who later were diagnosed with prostate cancer. Honestly, these men seemed more concerned about stopping their testosterone treatments than they were about the new diagnosis of prostate cancer. Some of these men chose their cancer treatment based on how quickly they could resume their TRT. After an extensive discussion regarding the risks and benefits, I offer prostate cancer survivors the choice to resume TRT one year after radical prostatectomy and 18 months after radiation treatment, if there is no more evidence of cancer.

It's difficult to say how long it will take before this medical question gets a full answer. In the meantime, if your partner is a prostate cancer survivor considering TRT, then schedule a serious discussion with your doctor about the rewards and risks of choosing such a path.

The three of you may put your heads together to decide that the quality-of-life side of the argument wins out over the risks you might be taking if you decide to have TRT. That would mean regular screening for the recurrence of prostate cancer. Or you may decide TRT presents too much of a risk for a recurrence of the disease. That would leave your partner suffering with, or trying to manage, the effects of Low T.

On the other hand, your doctor may tell you he is opposed even to considering TRT for someone who has fully recovered from prostate cancer. If that is the case, you will be faced with another decision: Do you take your doctor's advice and just forget about TRT, or do you seek a second opinion from another qualified medical professional?

Some strong evidence exists that it is safe to treat prostate cancer survivors, who also suffer from Low T, with testosterone. Still, it is not yet possible to assess the risk of such treatment. It may be that one day the fears of treating men who have fully recovered from prostate cancer will go the way of past fears that TRT caused a higher risk for prostate cancer in the first place.

CHAPTER ELEVEN

What About Getting Older?

The Effects of Aging on Testosterone Levels

We Americans appear to be aging quite well these days. As a whole, we're living longer than ever and the number of US citizens over age sixty-five is doing nothing but increasing. Most of that has to do with the "Baby Boomers," those born during the post-World War II years between 1946 and 1964.

As of now, almost thirty-seven million Americans are age sixty-five or older. That's about 12.8 percent of the total population; between the years 2010 and 2030, that percentage is expected to increase to nearly 20 percent. Of Americans over sixty-five, about 13 percent (around 5.1 million) are age eighty-five and older. That number is expected to increase to about 21 million—an amazing increase of 500 percent over the past sixty-five years.

OK, so a lot of Americans are getting a lot older these days. What does that have to do with the subject of this book? In short, it means that far more older men means far more sufferers of the sometimes miserable, devastating effects of Low T.

An estimated four to five million American men currently suffer from Low T (though I believe that number is on the low side), with only about 5 percent of them receiving treatment. With the rapidly increasing number of American men older than sixty-five (one estimate says that a man in the US turns sixty-five every sixteen seconds), those numbers are bound to increase.

As if getting older itself doesn't present some not-so-welcome changes!

What Happens When You Age (In Case You Didn't Know)

Let's begin with the positive. Getting older certainly has many benefits, especially the knowledge and wisdom that many years and a long life usually give to us. That's why one middle-aged man, when asked if he would like to return to the age of twenty-one, replied, "Only if I could take with me what I know now!"

Certainly doing wise things to keep yourself healthy—eating good foods, getting enough exercise, avoiding bad habits like smoking and drinking too much, and getting enough sleep—can have a positive effect on the aging process. It really is possible to slow down the ravages of getting older. Still, no matter how well you take care of yourself, your body *will* age and you *will* feel and see the effects of that aging.

If you think getting plenty of exercise and eating right will essentially eliminate the effects of aging, just think about some of the great athletes who have established themselves as true sports heroes over the past several decades. No matter how well they took care of themselves and no matter how "injury free" they managed to remain, a time came when all of them witnessed their bodies slowing down. They discovered that, regardless of their overall health, they couldn't run as fast, jump as high, or lift as much as they once did.

Think about the greatest athletes we've enjoyed watching over just the past few decades—Magic Johnson and Michael Jordan in basketball,

Emmitt Smith and Brett Favre (though he was a little slow in accepting it) in football, Wayne Gretzky in hockey, and Cal Ripken Jr. and Nolan Ryan in baseball. Each of these players was among the greatest who ever played their respective games—but there came a time when we had to say goodbye to each of them on the court or field of competition.

The same thing will happen with our current crop of superstar athletes. One day, even the most elite of them will come face-to-face with the fact that while their hearts and minds still want to compete, their bodies won't allow it to happen at the same level they managed in their teens, twenties, and early thirties. It's simply a fact of life.

Did you ever notice that there are no 100-year-old third basemen in the major leagues?

Chances are really good—overwhelming, actually—that you're not a professional athlete. But you, too, will see the effects of aging on your body. Your muscles will grow less firm and strong than they once were. You'll find it easier to gain weight (and more difficult to take it off). Your sex drive, as well as the ability to perform like you once did, will decrease. Your skin will develop tell-tale wrinkles and age spots, and your hair may turn a different color (OK, I'll say it: You may turn a bit gray!). All of your senses—hearing, sight, touch, and taste—diminish as you age.

As the process moves past middle age (the 40s and 50s), the consequences of aging can become more obvious, and sometimes more worrisome. Older men are at much higher risk for serious health issues such as heart disease, osteoporosis (though that is far more common in women than in men), various types of cancer (especially prostate cancer)—the list goes on. By some estimates, an average man loses from twelve to twenty pounds of muscle and two inches in height.

Aging has many effects on a man's mind and body, and most of them we don't exactly enjoy. But as the late comedian George Burns once noted when someone asked about having another birthday while in his nineties, "It beats the alternative."

Where Does Testosterone Fit In the Aging Process?

The effects on the body of aging are due in large part to factors like normal wear and tear, illness or injury, and genetics. Some people simply age better than others, and there's not a whole lot that can be done about that. Just the other day I saw an 87-year-old patient who looked more like 70. He was still sexually active and energetic and his T levels were the highest that I have ever seen, in the 800s.

So where does testosterone fit into the aging equation? While getting older doesn't necessarily mean you will suffer from the effects of Low T, it does put you at a much higher risk for a large dip in your testosterone levels.

In the overwhelming majority of my patients whom I have diagnosed with Low T, the primary cause is simple aging. There are many cases where injury, illness, or some genetic disorder has caused the problem (and those can happen at ages younger than you might expect), but I don't see those as often as the cases caused by normal aging.

To put it bluntly, the number one cause of Low Testosterone levels in men is age. To take that a step further, *all* men will experience dips in their testosterone levels as they age—and there is no lifestyle change, no herbal remedy, and no medical treatment that can completely change that fact.

As you read in chapter 8, a healthy lifestyle can keep your testosterone levels from dipping to levels your doctor would diagnose as testosterone deficient; but the bottom-line truth is that the older you get, the lower your testosterone levels will dip. And those lower testosterone levels will reveal themselves in a decreasing sex drive as well as changes in body composition (more fat, less muscle).

Some of the changes that come with aging are normal and expected. But when you throw an unhealthy and abnormally low testosterone level into the mix, you have symptoms that can go far beyond the normal changes one would expect in an aging man.

Lowered Hormone Levels in
Men and Women—How They Differ

It's important to understand the differences in age-related drops in hormone levels between men and women. While the two have similarities, the differences loom larger.

First, a woman is born with a finite number of eggs, stored in her ovaries. The ovaries also produce the female sex hormones estrogen and progesterone, which, like testosterone in a man, have many effects on a woman's body. When a woman's ovaries stop producing an egg every month, usually between the ages of forty-five and fifty-five, she experiences the condition called "menopause." At this time, the monthly processes of menstruation and ovulation stop, and her ovaries produce sharply declining amounts of estrogen and progesterone. Sometimes the production of estrogen and progesterone stops completely. A woman is usually diagnosed as "menopausal" after twelve consecutive months without a menstrual period.

A variety of symptoms have been associated with menopause, and their onset can be very rapid and severe. These symptoms can include hot flashes, heart palpitations, insomnia, mood swings, changes in the skin, depression, anxiety, panic attacks, urinary incontinence, increased body fat, and a decrease or loss of sex drive. Many of these symptoms resemble the drop in testosterone levels, and many can be reduced or eliminated with hormone replacement therapy.

Where men and women are different, as it relates to the age-related decrease in hormone production, is in the rate and severity with which it happens. A man's testosterone levels don't usually drop as rapidly or drastically as a woman's levels of estrogen and progesterone drop during menopause. A man's hormone levels usually peak in the mid to late teens and then begin to decline, slowly at first, in his mid to late 20s. Testosterone levels decrease fairly steadily through the 30s and then drop faster when he reaches his early 40s. Women's levels of estrogen and progesterone more or less fall off a cliff during menopause, while a man's levels of testosterone decline slowly and steadily through middle age, with an increase in the rate of decline as he ages.

While the drop or loss of female sex hormones during middle age is called menopause, a male experiences what has been called "andropause" or "male menopause" when his testosterone levels drop to below normal for his age, or falls more rapidly than they should. This usually happens in a man's 50s or 60s.

One other difference between the age-related declines of sex hormones in men and women is that women completely lose their fertility, meaning they can no longer conceive. It becomes a physical impossibility, since their bodies no longer produce eggs to be fertilized. Most men, on the other hand, never completely lose their ability to father children. Even the men whose testosterone levels decline more severely than they should, still produce sperm cells—and in nearly the same numbers as they did when they were younger, even though the sperm cells themselves are not as active and may sometimes be deformed. Most men can still father children well into their 80s, if they live that long. Do you remember the late actor Tony Randall? He fathered his first child at age 76!

Why the Drop In T Levels with Age?

Why does age cause a reduction in testosterone levels? What process causes this to happen?

While there could be many reasons for a man's decline in T levels as he ages, the primary cause appears to be the normal and natural decreased blood flow that occurs during aging. Most important is the blood flow to the arteries around and in the testicles. This decreased blood flow adversely affects cells in the testicles called the Sertoli cells and the Leydig cells. The main function of the Sertoli cells, named after the Italian physiologist Enrico Sertoli, is to produce sperm cells through a multi-stage process called spermatogenesis. This is why there may be a slight drop in the number of sperm cells produced *and* why those sperm cells may be less active or deformed.

The Leydig cells' main function, as we've seen, is to produce male sex hormones, including testosterone. As men age, the number of Leydig cells—named after the German anatomist Franz Leydig, who discovered them in 1850— in their testicles decreases, meaning less testosterone makes its way into their bloodstreams.

(A quick public service announcement: This is yet another reason why men should do all they can to keep their cardiovascular systems in as good a working order as possible, especially as they age. Blood flow naturally decreases with age, but a man who gets enough exercise, consumes a healthy diet, keeps off excess weight, and doesn't smoke stands a better chance of staving off severe losses in blood flow. That means more blood making its way to the tiny arteries flowing into the testicles, which means he'll have a better chance of keeping his testosterone levels at a normal level later in life.)

Another consequence of aging in men is the increased production of sex hormone binding globulin (SHBG), which reduces the effects and activity of testosterone in his body. SHBG is produced mostly by the liver, but also comes from the brain and the testicles in men (and the uterus in women). SHBG is one of several proteins in the body called "glycoproteins," and it is important in several processes.

SHBG is known for its tendency to "bind" to testosterone in the bloodstream, rendering the latter unable to enter the cells so it can do what testosterone does within our bodies. So, the more SHBG in a man's bloodstream, the less "free" testosterone the man has. And that means that even if the testosterone is being produced, it can't affect the cells in his body.

Testosterone: Great Medicine
But No "Fountain of Youth"

In the early 16th century, the Spanish explorer Ponce de Leon, then serving as governor of what later would be called Puerto Rico, heard many stories about a miraculous water source the natives called "the Fountain of Youth." The water's magical powers were purported to keep one young.

De Leon became convinced that the fountain flowed on an island called Bimini, and with the permission of Spain's King Charles V, he decided to set sail to look for it. Ponce de Leon never found the Fountain of Youth, or Bimini. He had to settle for beginning the first Spanish settlement on mainland North America in what would later be called Florida.

Ponce de Leon was hardly the first man who looked—in vain, as it turned out—for a gateway to extended youth and vitality. He also certainly was far from the last.

The battle against the effects of aging rages in the United States, where it has become a multi-million dollar industry. We Americans shell out billions of dollars for our pills, our potions, our creams, our gym memberships, and many other things ... all in the hopes of staving off the inevitable effects of growing older.

As we get ready to end this chapter, I suppose this is as good a time as any to explain something about testosterone replacement therapy that many people might not understand. TRT is *not* some kind of magical "Fountain of Youth" that raises a fifty-, sixty-, or seventy-something man's testosterone levels to what they were when he was eighteen. A sixty-five-year-old man on testosterone therapy isn't going to wake up one morning with the sex drive of a twenty-one-year-old (and won't his wife be happy to hear *that*). A fifty-six-year-old who hasn't darkened the door of a gym in fifteen years won't suddenly acquire the ability to build muscle the way a twenty-five-year-old can.

Can TRT restore *some* of the lost sex drive in a man suffering from Low T? Sure! Can it help him to achieve erections that, up until now, had seemed like faint memories? It's happened in my own practice. Can it help him to regain some of the muscle tone and vigor he's lost over the past decade or so? Absolutely! Can it improve his outlook, attitude, and temperament? No doubt!

But if you think that taking a dose of testosterone will have roughly the same effects as when Popeye eats his spinach, then you're going to be sorely disappointed. It simply doesn't work that way.

If, on the other hand, you're approaching the possibility of starting TRT in the hopes that it might help produce the physical and emotional improvements we've just seen, and if you're willing to give the medicine time to do its work, then you're probably ready to take that step. Remember the key to being the best that you can be mentally, physically, and sexually is having a healthy testosterone level.

Bimini? Nah. But you might enjoy the Bahamas a lot more than you would have before treatment. And so might your partner.

CHAPTER TWELVE

What if We Don't get Treatment?

The Longer-Term Health Risks of Low T

By now, you've probably grown familiar with the symptoms of testosterone deficiency—the sexual problems, the mood swings, the irritability, the loss of energy, and the general loss of a feeling of well-being.

But as serious and life-altering as those symptoms can be, the potential long-term effects of Low T are far worse—some even deadly—if the Low T sufferer doesn't seek medical help.

Low testosterone doesn't *just* affect a man's sex drive or ability to perform in the bedroom. It doesn't *just* affect his moods or his energy level. And it doesn't *just* affect his "mojo" at work or at home. It affects nearly every part of him—physically, mentally, and emotionally.

Why It's So Important to Get a Diagnosis *and* Treatment

It's important to understand that our bodies are a collection of systems and organs, all working together to keep us functioning and healthy. Each of our systems, organs, glands, and other body parts depend on one another to keep the whole body functioning properly. When one of those systems fails or stops functioning at capacity, then our entire body suffers.

Testosterone is just one of many essential hormones our bodies produce. It plays a huge role in how our bodies process protein and create muscle mass and bone density. It helps control our blood sugar and regulates cholesterol levels. It helps us maintain our immune system and helps us remain healthy mentally and emotionally. And, of course, it gives us our sex drive and ability to perform sexually.

The physical and mental effects of Low T you'll be reading about in this chapter are often very interconnected. In many cases, the cause-effect relationship between these conditions goes both ways. In other words, if you suffer from overweight or obesity, then you're likely to suffer from Low T; and if you suffer from Low T, then you're far more likely to become overweight or even obese. Many similar examples of the inter-relatedness of body systems could be named, but you get the idea.

For these reasons, you can't afford to see the symptoms of Low Testosterone as inconveniences or as obstacles you have to "manage" or "just live with." If you suspect that you or your loved one might suffer from Low T, get to the doctor as soon as possible before things get any worse.

Consider some of the possible consequences of untreated Low T.

Alzheimer's Disease

In 1906, a German psychiatrist and neuropathologist named Aloysius "Alois" Alzheimer identified the first published case of what he called "presenile dementia," which his colleague, Emil Kraepelin, later identified as Alzheimer's disease.

Alzheimer's disease is a progressive—and eventually fatal—disease of the brain that destroys brain cells and causes severe memory loss, as well as other severe problems with thinking, memory, and behavior.

Alzheimer's disease is the most common form of dementia (dementia is the term used to describe a cluster of symptoms, such as loss of memory, judgment, and reasoning, as well as changes in behavior, mood, and the ability to communicate). The National Institute on Aging estimates that approximately 5.1 million Americans suffer from Alzheimer's disease, which is the seventh-leading cause of death in the United States. As of now, while there are treatments for some of the symptoms of Alzheimer's, there is no known cure.

Alzheimer's disease is a cruel condition that impedes the patient's ability to think, to understand, and to remember. It also negatively affects the ability to make decisions. What once were simple tasks become very difficult. The memory loss usually starts with recent events and eventually causes the patient to forget long-ago events. The disease alters the patient's emotions and moods, and he or she may lose all interest in things they previously enjoyed. Eventually, the disease affects the person's physical coordination and mobility. In time, the patient loses the ability to perform simple, day-to-day tasks such as eating, bathing, and dressing without help.

Several studies over the past decade or so have found a strong link between the risk of Alzheimer's disease and Low Testosterone in men. The medical reasons for this connection are frankly complicated, but for the purposes of this book, I'll simply say that testosterone, or a lack of it, has a big effect on the brain—including the brain of aging men. One of those effects is an increased risk of Alzheimer's disease.

Clinical Depression

We've already seen that some men with Low T feel listless and fatigued, have low libido and energy levels, and may become more moody, withdrawn, and sullen. These symptoms are very similar—almost identical in some ways—to those of clinical depression.

This similarity has resulted in many men, who actually suffered from Low T, being diagnosed with clinical depression and being placed on anti-depressant medications without being checked for Low T. Meanwhile, the actual problem went untreated (actually, it may have worsened in some cases, because some anti-depressants may further lower testosterone levels in men who aren't producing enough testosterone already) and many of the symptoms remained.

Even though many men with Low T have received misdiagnoses of clinical depression, studies within the past ten years have shown a link between Low T and clinical depression. These studies have proven that Low T levels in older men may cause diagnosable clinical depression.

According to some studies, around 30 percent of men over age fifty-five have Low Testosterone levels, and the numbers rise to around 35 percent for men over age eighty. When men show signs of clinical depression, however, their testosterone levels rarely get checked, which leaves them vulnerable to the symptoms and other long-term effects of testosterone deficiency.

In a two-year study at the Puget Sound Health Care System and the University of Washington, researchers studied the medical records of 278 men over the age of forty-five who had no previous diagnosis of clinical depression prior to the study, but who had been diagnosed with normal to Low Testosterone levels. The men with Low Testosterone were found to be *more than three times* more likely to be diagnosed with clinical depression than other men.

The chicken-egg question about whether Low T causes clinical depression comes from the fact that the symptoms of Low T can profoundly affect mood or even lead Low T sufferers to bouts of depression. Other studies have shown, however, that Low T may directly alter brain chemistry, which changes due to aging anyway, leaving the elderly Low T sufferer vulnerable to clinical depression.

Either way, the evidence shows that men with Low T, especially the elderly, are *far* more likely to develop clinical depression than men whose testosterone levels are normal.

And the news doesn't stop there.

One of the major risk factors for suicide for people of all ages is clinical depression. Add to that the fact that older men have the highest suicide rate of any age group, and ladies, you have a very strong reason to get your partner's Low Testosterone diagnosed and treated—and sooner rather than later.

The symptoms of clinical depression can vary greatly from person to person. For some, it's obvious to everyone that something "just isn't right." In others, the symptoms may appear subtle or even hidden. Consider a few things to watch for:

- Feelings of sadness
- Crying spells
- Loss of interest in things the person once enjoyed
- Noticeable loss or gain in appetite
- Significant weight loss or gain
- Change in sleep patterns
- Agitation or irritability
- Fatigue or loss of energy
- Isolation from friends and family
- Trouble concentrating
- Feelings of worthlessness or excessive guilt
- Thoughts of death or suicide

If you can see these symptoms in yourself or in your partner, it's important to get medical help as soon as possible. And it is also a very good idea to check for Low T.

Heart Disease

At more than 615,000 deaths a year, heart disease is the single leading killer of Americans. When you consider the lifestyles of many Americans—their bad diet, their overweight condition, their smoking and drinking and lack of exercise—it's no wonder that so many people die of heart disease.

But here's a matter of serious concern for men who believe they may suffer from Low T (as well as the people who love them): There is a well-documented connection between heart disease and Low T.

In March of 2004, a study published in the Journal *Metabolism* held that Low Testosterone levels—not smoking, not high cholesterol, not diabetes, not overweight, not even high blood pressure—is the single greatest risk marker for clogged arteries and heart attacks in men. Another study, this one a United Kingdom study released in 2010, showed that men who already have heart disease are prone to dying at a much earlier age if they are also testosterone deficient. This should feel especially troubling to someone who suspects that her partner suffers from Low T because, as you read in chapter 8, obesity, diabetes, and high blood pressure are all risk factors for heart disease *and* for Low T.

Men tend to have much higher rates of heart disease than women. Once it was thought that the female sex hormone estrogen was the reason for the difference in heart disease rates. But new findings suggest that a normal, healthy level of testosterone helps prevent heart disease in men.

Men can do many things to reduce their chances of becoming a heart disease statistic: Lose weight, stop smoking, get regular exercise, and lower their blood pressure and cholesterol levels. As a medical health professional, I would encourage all men who are at higher risk for heart disease to do all those things. But it's also vitally important for men to get their testosterone level checked.

Anemia

As we have seen, anemia is a condition in which the body suffers a decrease in the number of red blood cells, or less than the normal quantity of hemoglobin. Red blood cells are responsible for carrying oxygen from the lungs to the tissues and organs of the body, and for carrying carbon dioxide from the body's cells back to the lungs. Anemia can lead to a condition called hypoxia (a lack of oxygen) in the internal organs, which can lead to a variety of medical problems, some of which can be deadly.

Anemia is the most common blood disorder and is one of the many potential consequences of testosterone deficiency in men. One of testosterone's many functions is to promote the production of red blood cells; so when a man's testosterone level gets low, his red blood cell count likely will dip, too. This is especially true of testosterone deficient men who also have type 2 diabetes.

Increased Abdominal Fat and General Weight Gain

We have seen that being overweight and obesity are big risk factors for Low T. The reverse also is true: Men with Low T are likely to become overweight or obese. The weight gain is often seen especially around the mid-section, the so-called "spare tire" many men develop as they age.

Metabolic Syndrome

Metabolic syndrome is a combination of medical disorders—high blood pressure, elevated insulin levels, excess body fat (especially around the waist), and abnormal cholesterol levels—that increase the patient's risk of cardiovascular disease, stroke, and diabetes.

Any one of the conditions listed above can increase a patient's risk of serious medical problems, and the combination of them can be very dangerous to his or her health. Even more frightening is the fact that metabolic syndrome affects between 20 and 25 percent of the population in the United States.

The risk of developing metabolic syndrome increases with age and with Low Testosterone levels. Men with Low Testosterone levels, especially the elderly, are far more likely to develop the syndrome. On the other hand, men with normal to high testosterone levels are far *less* likely to develop this syndrome.

Diabetes

Diabetes is a sometimes deadly disease that causes the patient to have high blood sugar—either because the body does not produce enough insulin (type 1 diabetes), or because the body's cells do not respond to the insulin the body produces (type 2 diabetes).

The medical community is somewhat divided on the relationship between Low T and diabetes. While there's no doubt that a close link exists between Low T and diabetes, the question is, does diabetes cause Low T (it certainly is a risk factor), or is it the other way around? Or does it work both ways? Men with diabetes are more likely to have Low Testosterone and men with Low Testosterone are more likely to later develop diabetes. No matter how this dangerous arrangement works, the fact is that close to half of all men with diabetes who are tested for testosterone deficiency are also diagnosed with Low T.

Among its many other functions, testosterone helps the body's tissues to take in more blood sugar in response to insulin. So when a man suffers from testosterone deficiency, he often develops a resistance to insulin (type 2 diabetes). This problem can cause several devastating physical problems, including cardiovascular disease and atherosclerosis, also known as hardening of the arteries.

Osteoporosis

The word *osteoporosis* literally means "porous bones," making it a fitting name for another condition associated with Low T. This condition occurs when the bones lose too much of their protein and mineral content (especially calcium), leading to a loss in bone mass and strength. This condition results in fragile bones that break very easily. In severe cases, even a cough or a sudden movement may cause the bone to fracture.

Fractures due to osteoporosis can affect any bone, with the most common breaks taking place in the hip, wrist, or spine. Fractures of the hips and spine can be very serious, as most often they require hospitalization and surgery. Such serious injuries can lead to permanent disability and even death.

By a large margin, osteoporosis affects women (usually postmenopausal women) more commonly then men. But lowered testosterone levels have been linked to higher incidences of osteoporosis in men, especially men over age sixty.

Osteoporosis develops more commonly in postmenopausal women because the female sex hormone estrogen helps protect women's bones from losing their density, and when women go through menopause, their ovaries stop producing estrogen. This situation leads to lower bone density and a substantial increase in the risk for developing osteoporosis.

Men's bones also are protected with estrogen, but in smaller amounts. As you may recall, small amounts of a man's testosterone are converted into estrogen inside his body. Therefore, when a man's testosterone level dips, so does his level of estrogen, which can lead to a weakening of the bones.

Testosterone replacement therapy is, along with increased calcium intake, an option for treatment for men with osteoporosis, and over time it can reverse the effects of osteoporosis.

The Bottom Line

Directly or indirectly, testosterone plays a big role, not just in a man's sexual health, but in almost every one of the bodily systems that work together to give him health. Without a normal supply of testosterone flowing through his veins, a man becomes susceptible to a wide variety of physical and mental ailments, some of them extremely serious.

This is why it is so important for any man who demonstrates the symptoms of Low T to see his doctor and get checked for this all-too-common condition.

But the question remains: Can receiving testosterone therapy help cure the diseases I've listed in this chapter, or at least help improve the patient's health in these areas? Sometimes the answer is definitely yes; at other times, probably no; and at yet other times, maybe.

Without question, however, Low T is not a medical condition you can afford to ignore. Left untreated, it can have disastrous effects on your health and well-being, and can even lead to potentially fatal health problems.

But as we've seen throughout this book, there is good reason for hope. A man with Low T isn't destined to die of a heart attack, or to develop anemia, diabetes, or any of the potentially serious consequences of Low T just listed. Help is readily available, and with a good combination of medical treatment and healthy lifestyle choices, a man with Low T has a great chance for recovery and a good chance to live a long, healthy life.

Why suffer with Low T when you can regain a life of high E (energy)?

CHAPTER THIRTEEN

Your Role, Ladies

Giving Your Support and Assistance for the Low T Sufferer in Your Life

What keeps most men from going to the doctor, even when their loved ones think they should? In my experience, the answer comes down to one word:

Pride.

I find myself constantly telling my children to "take pride" in their schoolwork, in their handwriting, in their appearance, and how they live their lives. That's the healthy side of pride.

But there's a negative side, too, that we might define as "the opposite of humility." This kind of pride is our enemy—it keeps us from venturing out of our comfort zone and seeking the help and answers we need, or from admitting (to ourselves and to others) that something is wrong. Pride could have kept us from writing this book. Wouldn't it have been easier just to leave our "messy stuff" in the dark?

Not for us.

Pride is the culprit that takes down marriages, friendships, families and individuals. All of us suffer from the damaging effects of this kind of pride, and I believe it's this sort of "I've got it all together, no matter what you say" kind of pride that keeps men from seeking the help they require. This kind of pride keeps men from asking directions, prevents them from admitting their shortcomings, and prompts many men to remain in denial over their health.

Why is this? I have a pretty strong hunch. When have we women ever had to prove our "womanhood?" Yet men feel as though they must prove they are a "MAN" every day. It must be exhausting for them! The same nuts in the media who tell us that we need to look like the airbrushed girls on fashion magazine covers are telling the men in our lives that they have to have it all together and never show any weakness. This is why most of us—wives, girlfriends, and significant others— are the ones who first nudge the men in our lives toward the doctor's office when we realize they are not themselves. Trust me, I have been the "nudger," and it is worth it.

Do not let fear of rejection or anger slow you down. Go for it! No matter how he reacts at first, deep down he will know that you are his partner—and that includes his health.

I know that what I am asking you to do is not easy. As I've said, I have been there myself. I have friends who have been there, too.

Are you there now? You know something is off with the man in your life; that is why you bought this book. I knew something was wrong with Sloan, but insecurity and fear kept me from seeking solutions. I felt too embarrassed to say anything to my husband, whom I loved, because I couldn't see what my part in it might be. I went through every possible scenario in my head: How could I have brought this on? Does he notice *that I have gained a few pounds? Maybe if I lost them, maybe then things would get back to normal. It affected every area of my self-confidence: Is it me? Is it my fault? Eventually, this self-doubt takes its toll.*

Confronting your husband about his sexuality is one of the most horrible things in the world for a wife to have to do. My friend did it; let's call her Katherine. Her marriage was failing and the two of them had not been intimate in over a year. If communication is not a strong point in your marriage—a real problem for my dear friend—this can become even more of a hill to climb. Katherine said it took her a year to get up the gumption to confront her husband, and he responded with a line of excuses: Work, stress, it went on and on. The denial continued, as did significant damage to the marriage.

In my opinion, trust breeds intimacy; and if you are not intimate, then trust drains away. After years of isolation, Katherine strayed and her marriage crumbled.

Honestly, in Katherine's case, her husband put off an exam too long. Only after the divorce became final did he find out that he had an extreme case of Low Testosterone. Now, I am not saying that Testosterone Replacement Therapy would have saved my friend's marriage; but I wish they would have known. When I told Katherine about this book and what Sloan and I were writing together, she felt thrilled. She and I agreed that it is critical to address these issues, both lovingly and persistently, before they permanently damage your relationship. Don't wait! Because deep down, he realizes it's time to find out what's up.

Lack of Knowledge

When members of older generations hear that a husband has lost interest in the bedroom, many give one of two answers: either he is having an affair, or he "plays for the other team."

I pray that now there will be another option: **Check his T level!** *Most men my husband diagnoses with Low T come to see him because of either a lack of energy or sex drive. Sloan has realized through his medical practice that not only do patients on Testosterone Replacement Therapy see improvement in those two areas, they also see improvement in many other areas of their lives, as well. Increased focus, motivation and enjoyment of life—and an improvement in overall mood—often result. Many guys didn't even know they were "off" there, but once they got them back, they felt thrilled.*

It is worth it! So make the effort, ladies.

It's a Matter of Teamwork

On my wedding night, my Dad gave me the best advice. He said that a good relationship isn't a 50/50 proposition—where each partner kicks in half of what it takes to keep the relationship healthy and growing—but a 100/100 arrangement where each partner gives everything he or she has to making their union everything it can be.

That's not just a good definition of teamwork in a man/woman relationship; it's also a good thing to remember as you and your partner do whatever it takes to help him recover from the effects of Low T. Why is that important, you ask? Because it may take that kind of teamwork as you and your man seek a diagnosis of his symptoms and begin the process—and make no mistake, it is a process—of recovery.

Here's a little fact that most women need to understand about us men (especially those of us who suffer from Low T): Most of us are naturally "wired" to desire and require the support and encouragement of the women in our lives. Sometimes we even need a little push to help us take the first step toward the road to recovery from the effects of Low T.

So consider several things you can do, ladies, starting with the attitude your partner will find most helpful.

Remember, It's Really Not about You

I've seen it many times in my practice, and it's something that needs attention here: Low T doesn't affect just the man who suffers from this condition, it also affects the woman in his life.

I find it hard to imagine how a woman who loves and lives with a man who suffers from Low T can't be adversely affected by his condition. After all, she's the one who lives with him, sleeps with him, eats meals with him, and she is the one person around whom he lets down his guard and is "just himself."

The symptoms of Low T can affect many, if not all, of the parts that make up the whole of your relationship. So when you feel tempted to ask, "What have I done or not done?" or "Is he in these moods because of me?" don't give up! Just be patient with him as he begins his treatment. Realize that it's just a matter of time before he becomes the same man you've always loved and enjoyed.

It's really not about you!

I realize that it's not always easy to remember that you are not, in any way, the cause of his symptoms (even though they certainly affect you)—and neither is "aging." It's important, however, to keep reminding yourself of this fact, especially if you want to give him the support and help he needs to overcome this condition.

He may seem depressed, lethargic, and tired all the time, but you didn't make him that way. He may seem a little irritable and moody, but nothing you've done or said caused that. And he may seem disinterested in sexual intimacy, but that doesn't mean you aren't attractive and desirable to him—or that he loves you any less.

To put it bluntly, if your husband has Low T, he's sick and in need of medical attention. And the more you can remember that fact and not lay the unpleasantness of the symptoms at your own feet, the more you can give him the loving support and help he'll need as he returns to health and wholeness.

Again, *it's really not about you!*

I stress this point because I know how easy it is to forget it, or to doubt it. And it's especially important to remember it in the sexual part of your relationship.

You're Still Desirable—Even When He's Not Interested

It really tore my wife up inside when she realized that I just wasn't interested in sex—even for the purpose of procreation. My sexual disinterest devastated her. We already had two boys, and Susan hoped to add a little sister to the mix.

Like many women, perhaps most, Susan initially thought that my lack of interest in sex had something to do with her. She wondered, Is it something I'm doing? Or is it something I'm not doing? We'd been married twelve years. We got along well and I genuinely enjoyed being with her. The attraction I felt for her never wavered. But because I suffered from Low T, I had neither the desire nor the ability to physically express my attraction to her. It had nothing whatsoever to do with her and her attractiveness, and everything to do with me and my malfunctioning body.

Some of those Low T-produced thoughts and feelings remained even after I was diagnosed and started a regimen to replace the testosterone that my body had stopped producing naturally. Like any loving wife, Susan felt happy that I had started treatment, especially when she saw that it made me feel better. But still, deep down, it bothered her that I needed injections in order for my sexual desires to return.

Susan had to deal with the same thoughts and feelings that many women have when their man suffers from erectile dysfunction (ED) and has to begin using prescription drugs in order to "perform." Women in this situation often wonder why they can no longer provide the stimulation their men need in order to achieve enough of an erection to have sexual intercourse. Many wives in this situation ask themselves—or their husbands—"Aren't you attracted to me anymore? Am I not pretty to you? Just tell me what I need to do, or stop doing, and I'll do it!"

As I've noted previously, Susan mentioned to me those same thoughts and feelings a few times early on; but in the years since I began receiving treatment, she's given more voice to what she was going through at that time in our marriage:

> *I thought, if it makes him feel better, great! But at the same time, it offended me that he had to take an injection in order to want to have sex with me. I thought, Why would he need a shot to be attracted to me? I look good and I'm fun to be around— yet he doesn't want to make love to me? It offended me, frankly.*
>
> *Looking back now, Sloan has been on Testosterone Replacement for many years, and sometimes it is hard for me to remember what it was like before treatment. Before, when Low T was new in our lives, its presence annoyed me. Now, my perspective is completely different. I look at his medicine just the way someone with any other illness would.*
>
> *We are in a routine and nothing about that tube of gel offends me now!*

Just as it's perfectly normal for a woman to wonder if her man's simple lack of ability to perform sexually has something to do with her, it's also normal for a woman to wonder if the symptoms of Low T she sees in her man are somehow her fault.

When you're married to a man who doesn't seem interested in sexual intimacy with you, who seems lethargic and tired all the time, who goes through what seem like unreasonable mood swings, and who doesn't seem any longer to have his "mojo," it's easy to start looking inward. After all, no one else (other than him, of course) is more affected by his condition than you are.

You may find it very difficult to accept that his mood swings, lethargy, fatigue, and lack of sexual interest have nothing directly to do with you. But you'll find it a lot easier to help him back to wellness and wholeness if you just keep reminding yourself that what you're seeing in him does not have its source in you or in your marriage. Yes, it certainly affects you, sometimes in very difficult and painful ways; and yes, it can be very hard on your relationship. But you are not the cause.

Remind yourself, too, that the problem is not that he's stopped loving you. Nor is it that he's no longer attracted to you. Never forget that testosterone plays a huge role in your man's sex drive, and when there isn't enough of the stuff coursing through his veins, his hunger for sex is going to diminish, and sometimes almost disappear altogether. This is a function of his medical condition, not an indication of any deficit on your part.

It bears repeating: Low T can cause drastic changes in your man's personality and sex drive. That's the bad news. The good news is that it's a medical condition that responds very well to treatment. By remembering these things, you can play a huge role in ensuring he receives the treatment he needs, and so get him back on the road to "getting better."

Offer to Go with Him to Visit the Doctor, However Many Times It Takes

You cannot know for sure whether your man suffers from Low T unless he sees a medical professional to discuss his symptoms. I suggest that, rather than just sending him off to get a checkup, you offer to go with him. He might refuse; but then again, he might not. Why not give him the option?

Visiting the doctor with your willing partner communicates how much you care about him and how important it is to you that he get better. It also means that you bring two brains, two mouths, and two sets of eyes and ears to the appointment with his doctor. Despite how his condition may have adversely affected you, you still bring an element of objectivity to the proceedings. You may have noticed important things about his behavior that have escaped his attention—important things, perhaps, for the doctor to know before he makes his diagnosis and prescribes treatment. In addition, you may hear and remember the doctor's words better than he can, especially since he might not be feeling all that well (isn't that why you asked him to see the doctor in the first place?). And beyond that, he might feel a little embarrassed to tell the doctor about some of his symptoms, especially the sexual ones.

(Just so you know, most men would rather chew on a wad of aluminum foil impregnated with used motor oil than talk to another person about their sexual problems. Why? I suspect that's a whole book to itself; for now, suffice it to say that it's a guy thing.)

Once the doctor has made a diagnosis of Low T, the three of you can talk about the various treatments available and discuss which one might be best for him. You also can discuss the possible side effects, how long it could take before you see significant improvement, and other questions you might have.

Encourage Him to Use—and Continue Using—His Medicine

The teamwork you foster in your relationship can greatly assist in the process of recovery as the man in your life begins receiving testosterone replacement therapy. At this stage you can play an especially big part in helping him reach the level of wellness and wholeness he enjoyed in his younger years. You can do this by encouraging—and even helping—him to take his medicine.

Consider a few things you can do:

Remind him to use his medicine. When your partner begins his testosterone replacement therapy, he's not going to stay home and wait until he gets better. He's going to continue his work life and other activities, both the ones he does by himself and the ones the two of you do together. A busy life can sometimes make it easy to forget or put off taking the medicine we need to get well! So it's helpful for him to have someone he loves remind him to take his medicine.

Make sure he keeps using the medicine, even after he begins feeling better. Once the full effect of testosterone replacement therapy begins kicking in, some men feel tempted to stop taking their medicine, or to reduce the prescribed doses. When the medicine takes full effect, he starts feeling better, maybe better than he's felt in years. He feels more energetic, the mood swings vanish, and he even starts getting that twinkle in his eye (you remember that twinkle, don't you?). At that point, he might start to believe, whether consciously or subconsciously, that the medicine has done its work and that he can stop using it.

Please make sure that doesn't happen!

Getting treatment for Low T isn't like taking a short series of antibiotics for a bad case of bronchitis, where you take a few pills or get a shot until the bronchitis clears up, and then the treatment stops. The man with Low T can't take a few doses and then expect that everything will be right with his body for the rest of his life. It's true that there have been a very few uncommon cases in which a man receives testosterone therapy for a time, his body gets a "kick start," and he begins producing more testosterone on his own. In the overwhelming majority of cases, however, if the Low T sufferer stops taking his medicine, his testosterone levels dip again and his symptoms return.

That's why the man who begins testosterone replacement therapy most likely will have to continue the treatment indefinitely, perhaps even for the rest of his life. So if you see any sign that he might want to stop taking his medicine, gently remind him, "Sweetheart, the doctor said you can't stop using the medicine." Of course, you're not his mother, but his partner and his teammate, so nagging won't help. Loving reminders, however, probably will.

Help him apply the medicine safely. I'm probably not far off the mark to say that most people, men and women alike, feel uncomfortable giving themselves injections. Who likes jabbing themselves with a needle? Your man could be different, but if not, you might want to consider learning how to give your partner the injections.

If you and your loved one decide to use the injection form of testosterone treatment, then you might get to "play nurse" every two weeks to give him the shot. It may take you a few times to get comfortable giving the injection, but the effort you expend can save you both the time and the bother of making and keeping doctor's appointments. Also, testosterone injections work best in the patient's behind; and even in his best days, your partner probably doesn't have the flexibility or dexterity to pull that off.

If the two of you decide with your doctor that testosterone creams or gels are the way to go, please remember that it is strongly recommended that women not come in contact with testosterone gels or creams. Avoid trying to apply these medicines for him; at the very least, not without rubber gloves. With this kind of therapy, you can be most helpful by consistently reminding him to apply these medicines as prescribed. The same holds true for patches.

Keep an eye out for possible side effects. Chapter 4 described the different forms of testosterone replacement therapy available today, as well as the possible side effects of each. If you or your partner begins to notice negative side effects from taking his medicine, please see your doctor so that adjustments can be made to the prescription.

Remind Him He's Still All Man … The Man You Love!

You don't have to be a big-time Beatles fan (though most Baby Boomers probably have a hard time figuring out how someone wouldn't like at least some of the Fab Four's music) to know this line from their mega-hit song "Yesterday":

Suddenly, I'm not half the man I used to be…

Men who suffer from the effects of Low T can relate to that line as well as anyone. Though the symptoms don't normally show up all at once, this feeling of being "less than I once was" often marks exactly how many Low T sufferers feel and think, especially before they know they suffer with the condition.

Maybe he doesn't feel as productive in his work as he once did. Perhaps he can't seem to find that "edge" that served him well for so many years. He knows he's been a bit on the moody and temperamental side, and that bothers him; he knows he isn't "that kind of person." And yet, he can't seem to get himself on an even keel. And his lack of sex drive? That's always what made him feel most like a man—and when that disappears, he wonders if he's lost an important part of his manhood. It's not merely that he can't perform as he once did; worse, it's that he doesn't even feel like performing!

One of the most important messages a woman living with a man with Low T can continuously communicate, through both words and deeds, is that *he isn't less of a man because he suffers from these symptoms.* He isn't less of a man because his sex drive has dwindled. He isn't less of a man because his energy levels have fallen. And he's not less of a man because his muscle mass and strength have dropped off to a place he dislikes.

Let him know that he's still the man he's always been, and that you love him and respect him and value him just as much as you always have. And then, let him know that you will do whatever it takes to help him get on the road to recovery and wholeness.

He'll need to hear those things from you. And he'll need to know that no matter how long it takes or what he has to do in order to recover, you'll be right there with him.

That's what love and teamwork are all about!

CHAPTER FOURTEEN

Q & A

1. **My doctor told me I have a normal T level, but I still have a lot of the classic symptoms of Low T. What should I do?**

   Make sure that your doctor checked both a free and total T and that he or she is using the normal ranges discussed in this book, and not the normal ranges listed on the lab report.

2. **Can I be diagnosed with testosterone deficiency, even if I have a normal to elevated total T?**

   Yes, if you are one of the rare men who have too much SHBG (sex hormone binding globulin) in your blood; then you could have an unusually high total T, but still a low Free T, and therefore a T deficiency that requires treatment.

3. **How do I prevent getting my T gel accidentally on my wife or children?**

   After you put on the gel, wash your hands with soap and water and put on clothing that covers the affected area of skin. After two hours, the gel is sufficiently absorbed into your skin and you (and your family members) should be safe.

4. **Does the time of day a blood test is performed affect the results in any way?**

No, the fluctuations in testosterone during the daytime hours is minimal. T levels will be highest in the early morning, but they shouldn't be so pronounced that they would affect a diagnosis.

5. **What are the benefits of being on testosterone replacement therapy?**

In my opinion, there is no way that a man can be the best he can be without a healthy T level. Having a T level in the normal range will optimize sexual, physical, and mental function, as well as maintain a healthy mood and energy level. With TRT, sleep improves for most men, too.

6. **What are the side effects of testosterone replacement therapy?**

The most common side effects are increase in body hair growth (unfortunately it doesn't affect hair growth on the scalp), increase in red blood cell count, slight elevation in PSA blood test, and increased appetite. These can be monitored by your physician, with the medication dose adjusted accordingly.

7. **Will TRT cause my man to become too aggressive or mean?**

This should not happen if his T level is not too high and in the proper range. If it does happen, then his T dose should be lowered. Sometimes at the very beginning of treatment, his levels may get a little high as his body adjusts. He may lose a little patience and be short tempered—but this is temporary.

8. **How long will I need to be on the medication?**

It is *highly* likely that you will need to remain on testosterone replacement thereapy for the rest of your life. Once you start using the medication, your body will produce even less T, since it is now getting the proper amount from another source. If you decide to stop the treatment for any reason, your body will again begin to make T, but your levels almost certainly will return only to their original, deficient level.

9. **Will my testicles shrink?**

Some men notice a slight decrease in size or fullness of their testicles after starting TRT. This is not harmful and just a sign that your body is relying on the medication.

10. **Does TRT cause prostate cancer?**

No, it is widely accepted that TRT does *not* cause prostate cancer *or* increase the risk of getting it. If anything, TRT will increase the chances of detecting prostate cancer, because men will undergo more frequent cancer screening during their course of treatment.

11. **Will I become bald if I start testosterone?**

No, TRT does not affect male pattern balding.

12. **How much does the prescription cost?**

Most insurance companies cover all forms of TRT, with a monthly co-pay anywhere from $30 to $100 per month. Injections are the cheapest form of TRT and cost an average of $30 per month, even without insurance coverage. Creams made at a compounding pharmacy can cost $30 to $75 per month, while gels cost $40 to $100 per month with an insurance co-pay; without insurance, they are very expensive, ranging between $250 to $400 per month.

Conclusion

The most recent data supports that Testosterone Deficiency effects 6% of the male population, it is also believed that 40% of men over the age of 45 suffer from Low Testosterone.

These statistics are alarming to us and we hope that with this book we will bring this condition to the forefront of everyday life. We have shared with you our personal story and also some of my patients so that you may understand the importance of a healthy testosterone level in men. By reading this book you have been empowered to discuss this with your loved one, or see the symptoms in your own life. As a medical expert and practicing urologist, I see the benefits of testosterone replacement therapy in myself and my patients every day. The successful treatment of Low T has a life-changing impact. So our point? Go get checked and know your T level.

Remember: the secret to a man's sexual, mental and physical wellness is a healthy testosterone level.

Author Biography

Sloan Teeple, M.D. is a Board-Certified Urologist and expert in Testosterone Deficiency. He is a partner at Amarillo Urology Associates, focuses his practice on Testosterone Replacement Therapy, and was personally diagnosed with Low T in 2004. Dr. Teeple trained in urologic surgery at Louisiana State University in Shreveport, Louisiana and attended medical school at the University of Texas Medical Branch in Galveston, Texas. He met his wife, Susan, while they both attended the University of Texas at Austin.

Dr. Teeple is an avid triathlete and completed his first Ironman competition in May 2011. He was raised in Austin, Texas and he and Susan now reside in Amarillo, Texas with their three children Chase, Hudson, and Evie.

Susan Morman Teeple was raised in Houston, Texas and attended The University of Texas at Austin and received her BA in African American History in 1994. Susan and Sloan have been married for 17 years and she has been a champion for Sloan during his medical education and training. Susan cares for their three children and enjoys running, cycling, and snow skiing. She is passionate about helping educate other women on the signs and symptoms of Low T, and share her story and experience with the disease.

Bibliography

1. "American Association of Clinical Endocrinologists Medical Guidelines for Clinical Practice for the Evaluation and Treatment of Hypo-gonadism in Adult Male Patients". (2002, Nov-Dec). *Endocrine Practice,* 8,6.

2. Coniff, R. (2007, Sept.). "Testosterone Under Attack". *Men's Health,* 182.

3. Crawford, E. (2007, October). "Hypogonadism and Testosterone Replacement Therapy: The Controversy and the Evidence". *Urology Times,* 1-10.

4. Cunningham, G. (2008, July). "Proceedings from the Testosterone Update. 1st Annual Conference on Improving Clinical Outcomes In Hypogonadism". *Grand Rounds in Urology,* 7,3.

5. Cunningham, G. & Shabsigh, R. (2007, March 10). "Testosterone Update. Bridging the Treatment Gaps in the Management of Hypogonadism". *Testosterone Update: Collaborative for Improved Clinical Outcomes in Hypogonadism.* 2007 Distinguished Faculty Meeting.

6. Gordon, E. (2006) *Testosterone Deficiency: The Hidden Disease.* New York. Universe, Inc.

7. Hellstrom, W. (2009, October). "Hypogonadism and Testosterone Replacement Therapy in Current Urological Practice". *AUA News,* 3-9.

8. Morgentaler, A. (2009). *Testosterone for Life: Recharge Your Vitality, Sex Drive, Muscle Mass and Overall Health!* New York: McGraw Hill.

9. Morgentaler, A. (2010, March). "Use of Testosterone therapy in Hypo-Gonadal men with Prostate Cancer". *Urology Times Clinical Edition*, 10-14.

10. Morgentaler, A. (2008, October). "Impact of Testosterone Deficiency On Men's Health". *Grand Rounds in Urology*, 7,5,6-11.

11. Nieschlag, E. (2004). "Testosterone Replacement Therapy: Current Trends and Future Directions". *Human Reproduction Update*, 10,5, 409-419.

12. O'Neill, B. (2005). *The Testosterone Edge.* New York: Hatherleigh Press.

13. Pope, H. (2003, January). "Testosterone Gel Supplementation for Men with Refractory Depression: A Randomized, Placebo-Controlled Trial". *American Journal of Psychiatry*, 160, 105-111.

14. Rosen, R. (2007, May). "Optimizing Testosterone Replacement Therapy In Hypogonadal Men". *Contemporary Urology*, 19,5.

15. Shippen, E. & Fryer, W. (1998). *The Testosterone Syndrome.* New York: M. Evans and Company, Inc.

16. Wang, C. (2000, March). "Pharmacokinetics of Transdermal Testosterone Gel in Hypogonadal Men: Application of Gel at One Site Versus Four Sites: A General Clinical Research Center Study". *The Journal of Clinical Endocrinology and Metabolism.* 85,3.

Printed in the USA
CPSIA information can be obtained
at www.ICGtesting.com
JSHW021433030724
65836JS00005B/232